HIKE LIST

P9-DMU-832

NASHVILLE

1   Anderson Road Fitness Trail (p. 14)
2   Bryant Grove Trail (p. 18)
3   Couchville Lake Loop (p. 22)
4   Ganier Ridge Loop (p. 26)
5   Harpeth Woods Trail (p. 29)
6   Lakeside Trail (p. 32)
7   Metro Center Levee Greenway (p. 35)
8   Mill Creek Greenway (p. 38)
9   Mossy Ridge Trail (p. 42)
10 Pinnacle Trail (p. 46)
11 Shelby Bottoms Nature Park: East Loop (p. 49)
12 Shelby Bottoms Nature Park: West Loop (p. 53)
13 South Radnor Lake Loop (p. 57)
14 Stones River Greenway of Nashville (p. 61)
15 Volunteer–Day Loop (p. 65)
16 Warner Woods Trail (p. 69)

WEST (including Ashland City, Clarksville, and Dickson)

17 Bells Bend Loop (p. 74)
18 Cumberland River Bicentennial Trail (p. 78)
19 Confederate Earthworks Walk (p. 81)
20 Dunbar Cave State Natural Area Loop (p. 85)
21 Fort Donelson Battlefield Loop (p. 88)
22 Henry Hollow Loop (p. 92)
23 Hidden Lake Double Loop (p. 96)
24 Highland Trail at Beaman Park (p. 100)
25 Johnsonville State Historic Area Loop (p. 104)
26 Montgomery Bell Northeast Loop (p. 108)
27 Montgomery Bell Southwest Loop (p. 111)
28 Narrows of Harpeth Hike (p. 116)
29 Nathan Bedford Forrest Five Mile Loop (p. 120)

SOUTHWEST (including Columbia, Fairview, and Franklin)

30 Burns Branch There-and-Back (p. 126)
31 Cheeks Bend Bluff View Trail (p. 129)

32 Devils Backbone Loop (p. 133)
33 Gordon House and Ferry Site Walk (p. 137)
34 Horseshoe Trail (p. 141)
35 Lakes of Bowie Loop (p. 144)
36 Meriwether Lewis Loop (p. 148)
37 Old Trace–Garrison Creek Loop (p. 152)
38 Perimeter Trail (p. 156)

SOUTHEAST (including Brentwood, Murfreesboro, and Smyrna)

39 Barfield Wilderness Loop (p. 162)
40 Brenthaven Bikeway Connector (p. 166)
41 Flat Rock Cedar Glades and
    Barrens Hike (p. 170)
42 Old Mill Trail (p. 174)
43 Old Stone Fort Loop (p. 178)
44 Short Springs State Natural Area Hike (p. 182)
45 Stones River Battlefield Loop (p. 186)
46 Stones River Greenway of Murfreesboro
    (p. 190)
47 Twin Forks Trail (p. 193)
48 Wild Turkey Trail (p. 197)

EAST (including Gallatin, Hendersonville, Lebanon, and Mount Juliet)

49 Bearwaller Gap Hiking Trail (p. 202)
50 Bledsoe Creek State Park Loop (p. 206)
51 Cedar Woods Trail (p. 210)
52 Collins River Nature Trail (p. 214)
53 Eagle Trail (p. 218)
54 Hidden Springs Trail (p. 222)
55 John C. Clayborn Millennium Trail (p. 226)
56 Jones Mill Trail (p. 230)
57 Old Hickory Trail (p. 233)
58 Peeler Park Greenway (p. 237)
59 Vesta Glade Trail (p. 241)
60 Wilderness Trail (p. 245)

MENASHA RIDGE PRESS
Birmingham, Alabama

60 HIKES WITHIN 60 MILES

NASHVILLE

INCLUDING
CLARKSVILLE, COLUMBIA, GALLATIN, AND MURFREESBORO

THIRD EDITION

JOHNNY MOLLOY

Library of Congress Cataloging-in-Publication Data

  Molloy, Johnny, 1961–
    60 hikes within 60 miles, Nashville : including Clarksville, Columbia,
    Gallatin and Murfreesboro / Johnny Molloy. — 3rd ed.
      p. cm.
    Includes bibliographical references and index.
    ISBN-13: 978-0-89732-848-7 (alk. paper)
    ISBN-10: 0-89732-848-5 (alk. paper)
    1. Hiking—Tennessee—Nashville Region—Guidebooks. 2. Trails—Tennessee—
    Nashville Region—Guidebooks. 3. Nashville Region (Tenn.)—Guidebooks.
    I. Title. II. Title: Sixty hikes within sixty miles, Nashville.
    GV199.42.T22N376 2010
    917.6804—dc22
                                          2009049589

Cover and text design by Steveco International
Cover photo © Dave Newman / iStockphoto
Author photo (page ix) © Lynette Barker
All other photos by Johnny Molloy
Maps by Steve Jones, Scott McGrew, and Johnny Molloy

Menasha Ridge Press
P.O. Box 43673
Birmingham, AL 35243
www.menasharidge.com

DISCLAIMER
This book is meant only as a guide to select trails in the Nashville area and does not guarantee hiker safety in any way—you hike at your own risk. Neither Menasha Ridge Press nor Johnny Molloy is liable for property loss or damage, personal injury, or death that result in any way from accessing or hiking the trails described in the following pages. Please be aware that hikers have been injured in the Nashville area. Be especially cautious when walking on or near boulders, steep inclines, and drop-offs, and do not attempt to explore terrain that may be beyond your abilities. To help ensure an uneventful hike, please read carefully the introduction to this book, and perhaps get further safety information and guidance from other sources. Familiarize yourself thoroughly with the areas you intend to visit before venturing out. Ask questions, and prepare for the unforeseen. Familiarize yourself with current weather reports, maps of the area you intend to visit, and any relevant park regulations.

This book is dedicated to the people of Nashville and Middle Tennessee, whether they are natives, transplants, or just came here to play music.

TABLE OF
CONTENTS

OVERVIEW MAP . . . . inside front cover

ACKNOWLEDGMENTS. VII

FOREWORD VIII

ABOUT THE AUTHOR IX

PREFACE X

HIKING RECOMMENDATIONS XIV

INTRODUCTION 1

NASHVILLE 12

1   Anderson Road Fitness Trail. 14

2   Bryant Grove Trail 18

3   Couchville Lake Loop. 22

4   Ganier Ridge Loop. 26

5   Harpeth Woods Trail 29

6   Lakeside Trail 32

7   Metro Center Levee Greenway 35

8   Mill Creek Greenway. 38

9   Mossy Ridge Trail 42

10   Pinnacle Trail. 46

11   Shelby Bottoms Nature Park: East Loop 49

12   Shelby Bottoms Nature Park: West Loop 53

13   South Radnor Lake Loop 57

14   Stones River Greenway of Nashville 61

15   Volunteer–Day Loop. 65

16   Warner Woods Trail 69

WEST (including Ashland City, Clarksville, and Dickson) 72

17   Bells Bend Loop. 74

18   Cumberland River Bicentennial Trail 78

19   Confederate Earthworks Walk 81

20   Dunbar Cave State Natural Area Loop 85

21   Fort Donelson Battlefield Loop 88

22   Henry Hollow Loop 92

23   Hidden Lake Double Loop. 96

24   Highland Trail at Beaman Park 100

25   Johnsonville State Historic Area Loop 104

26   Montgomery Bell Northeast Loop 108

27   Montgomery Bell Southwest Loop. 111

28   Narrows of Harpeth Hike. 116

29   Nathan Bedford Forrest Five Mile Loop 120

SOUTHWEST (including Columbia, Fairview, and Franklin) 124

30 Burns Branch There-and-Back 126
31 Cheeks Bend Bluff View Trail 129
32 Devils Backbone Loop 133
33 Gordon House and Ferry Site Walk 137
34 Horseshoe Trail 141
35 Lakes of Bowie Loop 144
36 Meriwether Lewis Loop 148
37 Old Trace–Garrison Creek Loop 152
38 Perimeter Trail 156

SOUTHEAST (including Brentwood, Murfreesboro, and Smyrna) 160

39 Barfield Wilderness Loop 162
40 Brenthaven Bikeway Connector 166
41 Flat Rock Cedar Glades and Barrens Hike 170
42 Old Mill Trail 174
43 Old Stone Fort Loop 178
44 Short Springs State Natural Area Hike 182
45 Stones River Battlefield Loop 186
46 Stones River Greenway of Murfreesboro 190
47 Twin Forks Trail 193
48 Wild Turkey Trail 197

EAST (including Gallatin, Hendersonville, Lebanon, and Mount Juliet) 200

49 Bearwaller Gap Hiking Trail 202
50 Bledsoe Creek State Park Loop 206
51 Cedar Woods Trail 210
52 Collins River Nature Trail 214
53 Eagle Trail 218
54 Hidden Springs Trail 222
55 John C. Clayborn Millennium Trail 226
56 Jones Mill Trail 230
57 Old Hickory Trail 233
58 Peeler Park Greenway 237
59 Vesta Glade Trail 241
60 Wilderness Trail 245

APPENDIX A—OUTDOOR SHOPS 250
APPENDIX B—PLACES TO BUY MAPS 251
APPENDIX C—HIKING CLUBS 252
INDEX 253
MAP LEGEND .... inside back cover

ACKNOWLEDGMENTS

I would like to thank many people for helping me with this project: Kelly Stewart and the Nashville Hiking Meetup Group, Pam Morgan, Dave Gilfillan, Lisa Daniel, Bud Zehmer (for coming up with the idea for the book), and Matt and Bailey Fields. I'd also like to thank Russell Helms, the rangers of Tennessee State Parks (including but not limited to John Froeschauer, Ben Myers, Tim Burris, Shane Petty, Amy Atkins, and Connie of Lebanon), the personnel at the Army Corps of Engineers lakes of Middle Tennessee, Natchez Trace Parkway. And thanks to Diane Manas of the Tennessee Trails Association and everyone I met on the trail.

—JOHNNY MOLLOY

FOREWORD

Welcome to Menasha Ridge Press's *60 Hikes within 60 Miles*, a series designed to provide hikers with the information they need to find and hike the very best trails surrounding metropolitan areas typically underserved by outdoor guidebooks.

Our strategy was simple: First, find a hiker who knows the area and loves to hike. Second, ask that person to spend a year researching the most popular and very best trails around. And third, have that person describe each trail in terms of difficulty, scenery, condition, elevation change, and all other categories of information that are important to hikers. "Pretend you've just completed a hike and met up with other hikers at the trailhead," we told each author. "Imagine their questions; be clear in your answers."

An experienced hiker and writer, author Johnny Molloy has selected 60 of the best hikes in and around the Nashville metropolitan area. From the rail trails and urban hikes that make use of parklands and streets, to flora- and fauna-rich treks along the numerous area lakes and hills in the hinterlands, to aerobic outings in the mountains, Molloy provides both hikers and walkers with a great variety of hikes—and all within roughly 60 miles of Nashville.

You'll get more out of this book if you take a moment to read the Introduction explaining how to read the trail listings. The Topo Maps section will help you understand how useful topos will be on a hike, and will also tell you where to get them. And though this is a "where to," not a "how to," guide, experienced hikers and novices alike will find the Introduction of particular value.

As much for the opportunity to free the spirit, as well as to free the body, let Johnny Molloy's hikes elevate you above the urban hurry.

All the best,
The Editors at Menasha Ridge Press

ABOUT THE AUTHOR

JOHNNY MOLLOY

A native of the Volunteer State, he was born in Memphis and moved to Knoxville in 1980 to attend the University of Tennessee. And in the nearby Smoky Mountains is where he developed his love of the natural world that has since become the primary focus of his life.

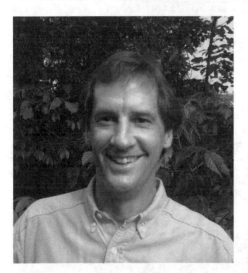

Molloy has averaged more than 100 nights in the wild per year since the early 1980s, backpacking and canoe camping in nearly every state in the nation. In fact, he has spent more than 650 nights in the lofty Smokies, where he cultivated his woodsmanship and expertise.

Now Molloy's love of the outdoors is a rewarding occupation. And the result of his efforts are more than 35 books, including hiking, camping, and paddling guidebooks; comprehensive guidebooks about specific areas; and true outdoor adventure books. Molloy has also written numerous magazine articles for Web sites and blogs. He continues to write and travel extensively, visiting all four corners of the country and endeavoring in a variety of outdoor pursuits. He is based in Johnson City, Tennessee. For the latest on Johnny Molloy, please visit **www.johnnymolloy.com**.

PREFACE

Welcome to the third edition of *60 Hikes within 60 Miles: Nashville*. The state of hiking in metro Music City continues to improve. New trails—included in this book—have been constructed and greenways expanded. Beyond hiking, Nashville is best known as the capital of country music and of Tennessee. Situated in the Cumberland River Valley and surrounded by hills of the Highland Rim, Nashville and its environs are nothing if not historic. In fact, most of the trails included in this guidebook have a historic bent, allowing visitors to walk both in nature and back in time.

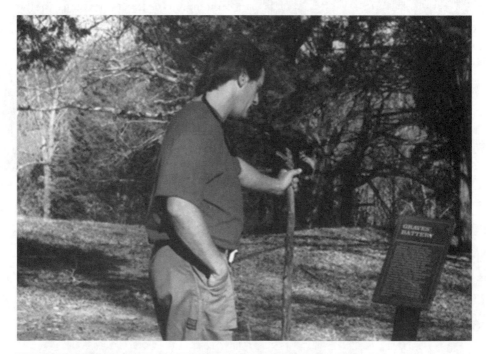

The author reading an interpretive sign along the Confederate Earthworks Walk

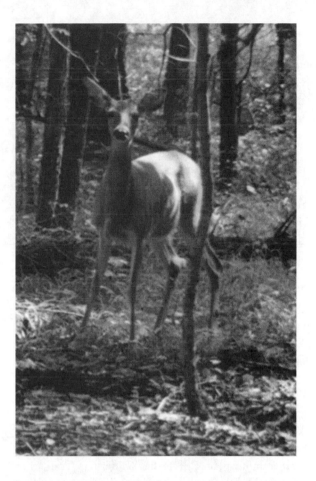

Deer on Wild Turkey Trail

Nashville's first citizens floated to the location on flatboats from East Tennessee. They headed down the Tennessee River, then up the Ohio and Cumberland rivers to reach the area that would become the city, which is located near a large riverside flat where Native Americans had been living for untold years. Simultaneously, long hunters (early pioneers who went on extended hikes) penetrated the basin from the east to find plentiful game attracted by the area's natural salt licks.

Early in its history, Nashville became the northern terminus of the Natchez Trace, a historic Native American trace, or trail, between the city and Natchez, Mississippi. In the early 1800s, boatmen walked north from Natchez after floating their crops and goods downriver from the Cumberland River Valley, the Ohio River Valley, and points north. Later, simple farmers settled in the Nashville Basin, opening what was then the west by clearing fields and building walls of stone that are now a Middle Tennessee hallmark.

Modern Middle Tennessee history begins in the Nashville settlement. Old Stone Fort State Park, near Manchester, houses a paleo-Indian site where the ancients built a wall. The reason it was built remains a mystery to this day. You can visit the wall for yourself and try to come up with a theory. And near Hohenwald, you can walk to the very spot where heralded American explorer Meriwether Lewis spent his last night on Earth at Grinder's Stand. There's evidence of the establishment of early Tennessee industry at Montgomery Bell's iron-forge site in Dickson County. And Johnsonville State Historic Area, to the west in Humphreys County, is the location of Nathan Bedford Forrest's unprecedented defeat of a naval force by a cavalry during the Civil War.

Dunbar Cave, up Clarksville way, held old-time hoedowns led by none other than country-music icon Roy Acuff. And other trails in Maury County preserve remnants of the original Natchez Trace built 200 years ago. You can walk these trails today and follow the footsteps of untold thousands who tramped by foot and horseback along Middle Tennessee's first "interstate," which is now preserved as a recreational hiking trail.

Some area parks have been created to memorialize both history and nature. The establishment of the Warner Parks and Radnor Lake State Park, for instance, recall stories of early citizen action aimed at preserving our natural heritage decades ago. Bowie Nature Park, near Fairview, tells the tale of three sisters who turned a worn-out family farm into a restored nature habitat.

Middle Tennessee is also laced with man-made lakes. Mostly built in the last half century, these impoundments were established for flood control and commerce on the Cumberland and Tennessee rivers' systems. These lakes have created recreational opportunities, such as boating, swimming, and fishing. With the establishment of Tennessee state parks and Army Corps of Engineers recreation areas on their shorelines, they also have become hiking destinations. Long Hunter State Park, on Percy Priest Lake, has many trails traversing the lakeshore and passing through interesting habitats, including rock gardens and cedar woods. Other areas, such as Newsome's Mill, were once settled and now preserve the relics of a former community.

The fast-growing Old Hickory Lake area has trails, too, such as the loop hike at Bledsoe Creek State Park that offers new residents nature getaways as Nashville expands ever outward. There are remote places, like the Wilderness Trail, that cover some of the roughest terrain in Middle Tennessee, along the steep shoreline of Cordell Hull Lake in Jackson County. And Fort Donelson National Battlefield stands tall on the shoreline of Lake Barkley, offering insights into Civil War battle strategies.

You can't forget the rivers. Tennessee's waterways have always been travel corridors, and now they're also hiking corridors. The Barfield Wilderness Loop travels along the West Fork Stones River. The Old Mill Trail bordering the Duck River explores a historic river ford used by Andrew Jackson and is the site of a corn-grinding station once run by a Tennessee governor. And the Narrows of Harpeth Trail climbs to a vista overlooking the lower Harpeth River. Smaller streams—such as Burns Branch on the Natchez Trace Parkway and Vaughns Creek on the Harpeth Woods Trail—are also worth exploring. And other untold, unnamed creeks can be seen and crossed on other hikes.

Of course, some areas have been established and preserved purely for their overall scenic or natural beauty. Short Springs State Natural Area is set aside primarily for its waterfalls and wildflowers. Flat Rock Cedar Glades and Barrens harbors rare plants unique to Middle Tennessee. Beaman Park preserves the oak ridges and steep-sided, wildflower-carpeted valleys of the Highland Rim. And the Devils Backbone State Natural Area preserves an intact hickory–oak upland forest with little intrusion from nonnative plants and animals.

Other trails have been established primarily for recreational purposes. The Anderson Road Fitness Trail allows area residents to stretch their legs in nature's gym; it offers good views too. The Couchville Lake Loop, a paved all-access trail resembling a running track, is utilized by walkers, runners, and those using wheelchairs. Jones Mill Trail, a new path at Long Hunter State Park, provides hikers and mountain bikers a way to burn some calories.

Then there are greenways, which Nashville and its surrounding communities all seem to be building to enhance the environs. Peeler Park Greenway and Metro Center Levee Greenway are two new additions to this edition. Stones River Greenway of Murfreesboro, which cruises alongside the Stones River, connects the town of Murfreesboro with Stones River National Battlefield. Shelby Nature Park travels beside the Cumberland River at a site not far from downtown Nashville. Cumberland River Bicentennial Trail traces an old railroad bed for miles along bluffs of the lower Cumberland River. And other greenways, such as the Stones River Greenway of Nashville, have been extended.

Finding all these trails became an exciting challenge. And walking them was a joy and a huge learning experience that I am grateful to share with potential readers. Being a native Tennessean, I was familiar with many destinations. Some (such as those at state parks) were obvious, but having written hiking and camping guidebooks about my home state alerted me to more. Being in the hiking world and frequenting outdoors stores helmed by knowledgeable employees helped too. Conveniently, while writing this book, I lived across the street from the Warner Parks, Nashville's premier in-town hiking destination. Including the hikes there was as easy as walking out the door. My feet also left an extra groove in the Harpeth Woods Trail.

Adding new hikes for this third edition was a challenge and a pleasure. I'll admit it—some places were duds that, after I hiked them, had to be eliminated from inclusion. But this book provides the service of doing the literal legwork of finding Nashville's best hikes and detailing them for the reader, including length, driving directions, scenery, facilities, related activities, and more.

This book will enable you to spend your precious time on the trail rather than finding a trail to get on. I sought to include destinations that had some outstanding feature, whether being historic, offering natural beauty, or featuring other activities you can combine with your walk. After hiking the trails included in this book, you too, I hope, will find something special about each one and see what a special place for hiking greater Nashville can be.

HIKING RECOMMENDATIONS

HIKES 1 TO 3 MILES

1. Anderson Road Fitness Trail (page 14)
3. Couchville Lake Loop (page 22)
4. Ganier Ridge Loop (page 26)
5. Harpeth Woods Trail (page 29)
6. Lakeside Trail (page 32)
8. Mill Creek Greenway (page 38)
12. Shelby Bottoms Nature Park: West Loop (page 53)
13. South Radnor Lake Loop (page 57)
16. Warner Woods Trail (page 69)
17. Bells Bend Loop (page 74)
19. Confederate Earthworks Walk (page 81)
20. Dunbar Cave State Natural Area Loop (page 85)
22. Henry Hollow Loop (page 92)
23. Hidden Lake Double Loop (page 96)
25. Johnsonville State Historic Area Loop (page 104)
28. Narrows of Harpeth Hike (page 116)
30. Burns Branch There-and-Back (page 126)
31. Cheeks Bend Bluff View Trail (page 129)
32. Devils Backbone Loop (page 133)
33. Gordon House and Ferry Site Walk (page 137)
34. Horseshoe Trail (page 141)
35. Lakes of Bowie Loop (page 144)
39. Barfield Wilderness Loop (page 162)
40. Brenthaven Bikeway Connector (page 166)
42. Old Mill Trail (page 174)
43. Old Stone Fort Loop (page 178)
44. Short Springs State Natural Area Hike (page 182)
47. Twin Forks Trail (page 193)
48. Wild Turkey Trail (page 197)
50. Bledsoe Creek State Park Loop (page 206)
51. Cedar Woods Trail (page 210)
53. Eagle Trail (page 218)

57. Old Hickory Trail (page 233)
58. Peeler Park Greenway (page 237)
59. Vesta Glade Trail (page 241)

HIKES 3 TO 6 MILES

 9. Mossy Ridge Trail (page 42)
10. Pinnacle Trail (page 46)
11. Shelby Bottoms Nature Park: East Loop (page 49)
14. Stones River Greenway of Nashville (page 61)
15. Volunteer–Day Loop (page 65)
21. Fort Donelson Battlefield Loop (page 88)
24. Highland Trail at Beaman Park (page 100)
26. Montgomery Bell Northeast Loop (page 108)
29. Nathan Bedford Forrest Five Mile Loop (page 120)
36. Meriwether Lewis Loop (page 148)
38. Perimeter Trail (page 156)
41. Flat Rock Cedar Glades and Barrens Hike (page 170)
45. Stones River Battlefield Loop (page 186)
46. Stones River Greenway of Murfreesboro (page 190)
54. Hidden Springs Trail (page 222)
56. Jones Mill Trail (page 230)
58. Peeler Park Greenway (page 237)

HIKES LONGER THAN 6 MILES

 2. Bryant Grove Trail (page 18)
18. Cumberland River Bicentennial Trail (page 78)
27. Montgomery Bell Southwest Loop (page 111)
37. Old Trace–Garrison Creek Loop (page 152)
49. Bearwaller Gap Hiking Trail (page 202)
55. John C. Clayborn Millennium Trail (page 226)
60. Wilderness Trail (page 245)

HIKES GOOD FOR YOUNG CHILDREN

 1. Anderson Road Fitness Trail (page 14)
 3. Couchville Lake Loop (page 22)
 8. Mill Creek Greenway (page 38)
12. Shelby Bottoms Nature Park: West Loop (page 53)
33. Gordon House and Ferry Site Walk (page 137)
34. Horseshoe Trail (page 141)
35. Lakes of Bowie Loop (page 144)
42. Old Mill Trail (page 174)
57. Old Hickory Trail (page 233)

CITY HIKES

4. Ganier Ridge Loop (page 26)
5. Harpeth Woods Trail (page 29)
7. Metro Center Levee Greenway (page 35)
8. Mill Creek Greenway (page 38)
14. Stones River Greenway of Nashville (page 61)
19. Confederate Earthworks Walk (page 81)
21. Fort Donelson Battlefield Loop (page 88)
22. Henry Hollow Loop (page 92)
25. Johnsonville State Historic Area Loop (page 104)
29. Nathan Bedford Forrest Five Mile Loop (page 120)
37. Old Trace–Garrison Creek Loop (page 152)
43. Old Stone Fort Loop (page 178)
44. Short Springs State Natural Area Hike (page 182)
46. Stones River Greenway of Murfreesboro (page 190)
55. John C. Clayborn Millennium Trail (page 226)
60. Wilderness Trail (page 245)

LAKE HIKES

2. Bryant Grove Trail (page 18)
3. Couchville Lake Loop (page 22)
15. Volunteer–Day Loop (page 65)
35. Lakes of Bowie Loop (page 144)
47. Twin Forks Trail (page 193)
50. Bledsoe Creek State Park Loop (page 206)
55. John C. Clayborn Millennium Trail (page 226)
56 Jones Mill Trail (page 230)
60. Wilderness Trail (page 245)

SCENIC HIKES

2. Bryant Grove Trail (page 18)
9. Mossy Ridge Trail (page 42)
15. Volunteer–Day Loop (page 65)
16. Warner Woods Trail (page 69)
18. Cumberland River Bicentennial Trail (page 78)
23. Hidden Lake Double Loop (page 96)
28. Narrows of Harpeth Hike (page 116)
30. Burns Branch There-and-Back (page 126)
31. Cheeks Bend Bluff View Trail (page 129)
41. Flat Rock Cedar Glades and Barrens Hike (page 170)
43. Old Stone Fort Loop (page 178)
44. Short Springs State Natural Area Hike (page 182)

53. Eagle Trail (page 218)
55. John C. Clayborn Millennium Trail (page 226)
60. Wilderness Trail (page 245)

HISTORIC HIKES

5. Harpeth Woods Trail (page 29)
12. Shelby Bottoms Nature Park: West Loop (page 53)
19. Confederate Earthworks Walk (page 81)
20. Dunbar Cave State Natural Area Loop (page 85)
21. Fort Donelson Battlefield Loop (page 88)
25. Johnsonville State Historic Area Loop (page 104)
27. Montgomery Bell Southwest Loop (page 111)
28. Narrows of Harpeth Hike (page 116)
33. Gordon House and Ferry Site Walk (page 137)
36. Meriwether Lewis Loop (page 148)
37. Old Trace–Garrison Creek Loop (page 152)
42. Old Mill Trail (page 174)
43. Old Stone Fort Loop (page 178)
45. Stones River Battlefield Loop (page 186)
46. Stones River Greenway of Murfreesboro (page 190)

HIKES FOR WILDLIFE VIEWING

17. Bells Bend Loop (page 74)
20. Dunbar Cave State Natural Area Loop (page 85)
22. Henry Hollow Loop (page 92)
24. Highland Trail at Beaman Park (page 100)
48. Wild Turkey Trail (page 197)
50. Bledsoe Creek State Park Loop (page 206)
54. Hidden Springs Trail (page 222)
57. Old Hickory Trail (page 233)

HIKES FOR WILDFLOWERS

13. South Radnor Lake Loop (page 57)
22. Henry Hollow Loop (page 92)
32. Devils Backbone Loop (page 133)
41. Flat Rock Cedar Glades and Barrens Hike (page 170)
43. Old Stone Fort Loop (page 178)
44. Short Springs State Natural Area Hike (page 182)
53. Eagle Trail (page 218)
56. Jones Mill Trail (page 230)
59. Vesta Glade Trail (page 241)

TRAILS FOR RUNNERS

7. Metro Center Levee Greenway (page 35)
8. Mill Creek Greenway (page 38)
14. Stones River Greenway of Nashville (page 61)
18. Cumberland River Bicentennial Trail (page 78)
40. Brenthaven Bikeway Connector (page 166)
46. Stones River Greenway of Murfreesboro (page 190)

TRAILS FOR BICYCLISTS

6. Lakeside Trail (page 32)
7. Metro Center Levee Greenway (page 35)
10. Pinnacle Trail (page 46)
14. Stones River Greenway of Nashville (page 61)
18. Cumberland River Bicentennial Trail (page 78)
38. Perimeter Trail (page 156)
40. Brenthaven Bikeway Connector (page 166)
46. Stones River Greenway of Murfreesboro (page 190)

LESS-BUSY HIKES

29. Nathan Bedford Forrest Five Mile Loop (page 120)
32. Devils Backbone Loop (page 133)
34. Horseshoe Trail (page 141)
37. Old Trace–Garrison Creek Loop (page 152)
41. Flat Rock Cedar Glades and Barrens Hike (page 170)
44. Short Springs State Natural Area Hike (page 182)
49. Bearwaller Gap Hiking Trail (page 202)
59. Vesta Glade Trail (page 241)
60. Wilderness Trail (page 245)

HEAVILY TRAVELED HIKES

4. Ganier Ridge Loop (page 26)
5. Harpeth Woods Trail (page 29)
13. South Radnor Lake Loop (page 57)
14. Stones River Greenway of Nashville (page 61)
46. Stones River Greenway of Murfreesboro (page 190)
56. Jones Mill Trail (page 230)

60 HIKES
WITHIN 60 MILES

NASHVILLE
INCLUDING
CLARKSVILLE, COLUMBIA, GALLATIN, AND MURFREESBORO

INTRODUCTION

Welcome to *60 Hikes within 60 Miles: Nashville!* If you're new to hiking, or even if you're a seasoned trailsmith, take a few minutes to read the following introduction. We'll explain how this book is organized and how to get the best use of it.

THE MAPS

THE OVERVIEW MAP AND MAP KEY

Use the overview map on the inside front cover to assess the exact location of each hike's primary trailhead. Each hike's number appears on the overview map, on the map key facing the overview map, and in the table of contents. Flipping through the book, you will easily locate a hike's full profile by watching for the hike number at the top of each page.

The book is organized by region, as indicated in the table of contents. A map legend that details the symbols found on the trail maps can be found on the inside back cover.

TRAIL MAPS

Each hike contains a detailed map that shows the trailhead, the route, significant features, facilities, and topographic landmarks such as creeks, overlooks, and peaks. Each trailhead's GPS coordinates are included with each profile.

GPS TRAILHEAD COORDINATES

This book includes GPS coordinates for each trailhead in two formats: latitude–longitude and UTM (Universal Transverse Mercator). Latitude–longitude coordinates tell you where you are by locating a point west (latitude) of the 0° meridian line that passes through Greenwich, England, and north or south (longitude) of the 0° line that belts the Earth, aka the Equator.

Topographic maps show latitude–longitude as well as UTM grid lines. Known as UTM coordinates, the numbers

1

index a specific point using a grid method. The survey datum used to arrive at the coordinates in this book is WGS84 (versus NAD27 or WGS83). For readers who own a GPS unit, whether handheld or onboard a vehicle, the latitude–longitude or UTM coordinates provided on the first page of each hike may be entered into the GPS unit. Just make sure your GPS unit is set to navigate using WGS84 datum. Now you can navigate directly to the trailhead.

Most trailheads, which begin in parking areas, can be reached by car, but some hikes still require a short walk to reach the trailhead from a parking area. In those cases a handheld unit is necessary to continue the GPS navigation process. That said, however, readers can easily access all trailheads in this book by using the directions given, the overview map, and the trail map, which shows at least one major road leading into the area. But for those who enjoy using the latest GPS technology to navigate, the necessary data has been provided. A brief explanation of the UTM coordinates from Hike 1, Anderson Road Fitness Trail (page 14), follows:

UTM Zone (WGS 84) 16S
Easting   0535919
Northing   3995737

The UTM zone number **16** refers to one of the 60 vertical zones of the UTM projection. Each zone is 6 degrees wide. The UTM zone letter **S** refers to one of the 20 horizontal zones that span from 80 degrees South to 84 degrees North. The easting number **0535919** indicates in meters how far east or west a point is from the central meridian of the zone. Increasing easting coordinates on a topo map or on your GPS screen indicate that you are moving east; decreasing easting coordinates indicate you are moving west. The northing number **3995737** references in meters how far you are from the equator. Above and below the equator, increasing northing coordinates indicate you are traveling north; decreasing northing coordinates indicate you are traveling south. To learn more about how to enhance your outdoor experiences with GPS technology, refer to *GPS Outdoors: A Practical Guide for Outdoor Enthusiasts* (Menasha Ridge Press).

HIKE DESCRIPTIONS

Each hike profile contains seven key items: a brief description of the trail, a Key At-a-Glance Information box, GPS coordinates, directions to the trailhead, a trail map, a hike description, and information on nearby activities when applicable. Combined, the maps and information provide a clear method to assess each trail from the comfort of your favorite reading chair.

IN BRIEF

A "taste of the trail." Think of this section as a snapshot focused on the historical landmarks, beautiful vistas, and other sights you may encounter on the trail.

KEY AT-A-GLANCE INFORMATION

The information boxes give you a quick idea of the specifics of each hike. There are 12 basic elements covered.

LENGTH   Options are often provided to shorten or extend the hikes, but the mileage corresponds to the described hike. Consult the hike description to decide how to customize the hike for your ability or time constraints.

CONFIGURATION   A description of what the trail might look like from overhead. Trails can be loops, out-and-backs (that is, along the same route), figure eights, or balloons. Sometimes the descriptions might surprise you.

DIFFICULTY   The degree of effort an average hiker should expect on a given hike. For simplicity, difficulty is described as "easy," "moderate," or "difficult."

SCENERY   A summary of the overall environs of the hike and what to expect in terms of plant life, wildlife, streams, and historic buildings.

EXPOSURE   A quick check of how much sun you can expect on your shoulders during the hike. Descriptors used are self-explanatory and include terms such as shady, exposed, and sunny.

TRAFFIC   Indicates how busy the trail might be on an average day and if you might be able to find solitude out there. Trail traffic, of course, varies from day to day and season to season.

TRAIL SURFACE   Indicates whether the trail is paved, rocky, smooth dirt, or a mixture of elements.

HIKING TIME   How long it took the author to hike the trail. Estimated times are based on an average pace of 2 to 3 mph, adjusted for the ease or difficulty of the hike's terrain. Hikes with widely ranging time estimates describe trail networks with hiking options of varying lengths. Keep in mind that if you're a birder, wildflower lover, amateur geologist, or a doze-on-rocks type like the author, hike times will be quite a bit longer.

ACCESS   Notes time of day when hike route is open, days when it is closed, and when permits or fees are needed to access the trail. When possible, directions to hikes begin from the nearest interstate exit off highways leading from Nashville. Directions to trails far from expressways start from nearby towns or major highway intersections.

MAPS   Which map is the best, or easiest to read (in the author's opinion) for this hike, and where to get it.

FACILITIES   What to expect in terms of restrooms, phones, water, and other niceties available at the trailhead or nearby.

SPECIAL COMMENTS   Provides you with those extra details that don't fit into any of the above categories. Here you'll find information on trail hiking options and facts such as whether or not to expect a lifeguard at a nearby swimming beach.

DIRECTIONS TO THE TRAIL

Used with the locator map, the directions will help you locate each trailhead.

TRAIL DESCRIPTIONS

The trail description is the heart of each hike. Here, the author provides a summary of the trail's essence, as well as a highlight of any special traits the hike offers. Ultimately, the hike description will help you choose which hikes are best for you.

NEARBY ACTIVITIES

Not every hike will have this listing. For those that do, look here for information on nearby sights of interest.

WEATHER

While any time is fine for hiking in the Nashville area, spring and fall are most folks' favorite seasons. The first warm breath of spring brings wildflowers, and seasonal rains bring the streams to life—waterfalls and cascades are everywhere in April and May. October brings spectacular fall colors, along with crisp, cool days free of bugs and humidity.

Winter is my favorite time to hike: no bugs, no heat or humidity, and best of all, no foliage. Vistas obscured by greenery in the warm months open up in winter, and when it's really cold, the streams, waterfalls, and seeps create incredible ice formations. Summer, with its heat and humidity, is a tough time to hike around Nashville. Get out early in the morning, or try something really unique— choose a park open after sunset and hike by the light of the full moon.

DAILY AVERAGE TEMPERATURES BY MONTH (degrees Fahrenheit)

	JAN	FEB	MAR	APR	MAY	JUN
MIN	21° F	27° F	36° F	47° F	57° F	66° F
MAX	38° F	44° F	55° F	67° F	77° F	85° F
MEAN	30° F	35° F	46° F	57° F	67° F	76° F
	JUL	AUG	SEP	OCT	NOV	DEC
MIN	71° F	69° F	60° F	48° F	37° F	26° F
MAX	90° F	88° F	80° F	68° F	54° F	42° F
MEAN	80° F	78° F	70° F	56° F	45° F	34° F

WATER

How much is enough? Well, one simple physiological fact should convince you to err on the side of excess when deciding how much water to pack: A hiker working hard in 90-degree heat needs approximately 10 quarts of fluid per day. That's 2.5 gallons—12 large water bottles or 16 small ones. In other words, pack along one or two bottles even for short hikes.

Some hikers and backpackers hit the trail prepared to purify water found along the route. This method, while less dangerous than drinking untreated water, comes with risks. Purifiers with ceramic filters are the safest. Many hikers pack along the slightly distasteful tetraglycine-hydroperiodide tablets (sold under the names Potable Aqua, Coughlan's, and others) to de-bug water.

Probably the most common waterborne "bug" that hikers face is *Giardia*, which may not hit until one to four weeks after ingestion. It will have you living in the bathroom, passing noxious rotten-egg gas, vomiting, and shivering with chills. Other parasites to worry about include *E. coli* and *Cryptosporidium*, both of which are harder to kill than *Giardia*.

For most people, the pleasures of hiking make carrying water a relatively minor price to pay to remain healthy. If you are tempted to drink "found water," do so only if you understand the risks involved. Better yet, hydrate prior to your hike, carry (and drink) 6 ounces of water for every mile you plan to hike, and hydrate again after the hike.

THE TEN ESSENTIALS

One of the first rules of hiking is to be prepared for anything. The simplest way to be prepared is to carry the "Ten Essentials," listed below. In addition to carrying them, you need to know how to use them, especially navigation items. Always consider worst-case scenarios like getting lost, hiking back in the dark, having broken gear (for example, a broken hip strap on your pack or a plugged water filter), twisting an ankle, or a brutal thunderstorm. The items listed below don't cost a lot of money, don't take up much room in a pack, and don't weigh much, but they might just save your life.

Water: durable bottles and water treatment like iodine or a filter

Maps: preferably a topographic map and a trail map that includes a route description

Compass: a high-quality compass

First-aid kit: a good-quality kit including first-aid instructions

Knife: a multitool device with pliers

Light: flashlight or headlamp with extra bulbs and batteries

Fire: windproof matches or a lighter and fire starter

Extra food: you should always have food in your pack when you've finished hiking

Extra clothes: rain protection, warm layers, gloves, warm hat

Sun protection: sunglasses, lip balm, sunblock, sun hat

FIRST-AID KIT

A typical first-aid kit may contain more items than you might think necessary. The list of supplies on the following page covers just the basics. Prepackaged kits in waterproof bags (Atwater Carey and Adventure Medical make a variety of kits) are also available. Even though quite a few items are listed here, they pack down into a small space:

- Ace bandages or Spenco joint wraps
- Antibiotic ointment (Neosporin or the generic equivalent)
- Aspirin or acetaminophen
- Band-Aids
- Benadryl or the generic equivalent—diphenhydramine (an antihistamine, in case of allergic reactions)
- Butterfly-closure bandages
- Epinephrine in a prefilled syringe (for those known to have severe allergic reactions to such things as bee stings)
- Gauze (one roll)
- Gauze compress pads (a half dozen 4-inch by 4-inch)
- Hydrogen peroxide or iodine
- Insect repellent
- Matches or pocket lighter
- Moleskin/Spenco "Second Skin"
- Snakebite kit
- Sunscreen
- Water-purification tablets or water filter (on longer hikes)
- Whistle (more effective in signaling rescuers than your voice)

TOPO MAPS

The maps in this book have been produced with great care and, used with the hiking directions, will direct you to the trail and help you stay on course. However, you will find superior detail and valuable information in the U.S. Geological Survey's 7.5-minute series topographic maps. Topo maps are available online in many locations. A well-known free service is at **www.terraserver.microsoft.com,** and another free service with fast click-and-drag browsing is at **www.topofinder.com.** You can view and print topos of the entire United States from these Web sites and view aerial photographs of the same area at Terraserver. Several online services such as **www.trails.com** charge annual fees for additional features such as shaded relief, which makes the topography stand out more. If you expect to print out many topo maps each year, it might be worth paying for shaded-relief topo maps. The downside to USGS topos is that most of them are outdated, having been created 20 to 30 years ago. But they still provide excellent topographic detail.

If you're new to hiking, you might be wondering, "What's a topographic map?" In short, a topo indicates not only linear distance but elevation as well, using contour lines. Contour lines spread across the map like dozens of intricate spider webs. Each line represents a particular elevation, and at the base of each topo, a contour's interval designation is given. If the contour interval is 20 feet, then the distance between each contour line is 20 feet. Follow five contour lines up on the same map, and the elevation has increased by 100 feet.

Let's assume that the 7.5-minute series topo reads "Contour Interval 40 feet," that the short trail we'll be hiking is 2 inches in length on the map, and that it crosses five contour lines from beginning to end. What do we know? Well, because the linear scale of this series is 2,000 feet to the inch (roughly 2.75 inches representing 1 mile), we know our trail is approximately 0.8 miles long (2 inches equals 2,000 feet). But we also know we'll be climbing or descending 200 vertical feet (five contour lines are 40 feet each) over that distance. And the elevation designations written on occasional contour lines will tell us if we're heading up or down.

In addition to the outdoor shops listed in the Appendix, you'll find topos at major universities and some public libraries, where you might try photocopying the ones you need to avoid the cost of buying them. But if you want your own and can't find them locally, visit the U.S. Geological Survey's Web site at **topomaps.usgs.gov.**

HIKING WITH CHILDREN

No one is too young for a hike in the outdoors. Be mindful, though. Flat, short, and shaded trails are best with an infant. Toddlers who have not quite mastered walking can still tag along, riding on an adult's back in a child carrier. Use common sense to judge a child's capacity to hike a particular trail, and always count that the child will tire quickly and need to be carried.

When packing for the hike, remember the child's needs as well as your own. Make sure children are adequately clothed for the weather, have proper shoes, and are protected from the sun with sunscreen. Kids dehydrate quickly, so make sure you have plenty of fluid for everyone. To assist an adult with determining which trails are suitable for youngsters, a list of hike recommendations for children is provided on page xv.

GENERAL SAFETY

No doubt, potentially dangerous situations can occur outdoors, but as long as you use sound judgment and prepare yourself before hitting the trail, you'll be safer in the woods than in most urban areas of the country. It is better to look at a backcountry hike as a fascinating chance to discover the unknown rather than a chance for potential disaster. Here are a few tips to make your trip safer and easier.

- **Always carry food and water whether you are planning to go overnight or not. Food will give you energy, help keep you warm, and sustain you in an emergency situation until help arrives. You never know if you will have a stream nearby when you become thirsty. Bring potable water or treat water before drinking it from a stream. Boil or filter all found water before drinking it.**

- **Stay on designated trails. Most hikers get lost when they leave the path. Even on the most clearly marked trails, there is usually a point where you have to stop and consider which direction to head. If you become disoriented, don't panic. As soon as you think you may be off track, stop, assess your current direction, and then retrace your steps back to the point where you went awry. Using map, compass, this book,** and keeping in mind what you have passed thus far, reorient yourself and trust your judgment on which way to continue. If you become absolutely unsure of how to continue, return to your vehicle the way you came in. Should you become completely lost and have no idea of how to return to the trailhead, remaining in place along the trail and waiting for help is most often the best option for adults and always the best option for children.

- Be especially careful when crossing streams. Whether you are fording the stream or crossing on a log, make every step count. If you have any doubt about maintaining your balance on a foot log, go ahead and ford the stream instead. When fording a stream, use a trekking pole or stout stick for balance and face upstream as you cross. If a stream seems too deep to ford, turn back. Whatever is on the other side is not worth risking your life.

- Be careful at overlooks. While these areas may provide spectacular views, they are potentially hazardous. Stay back from the edge of outcrops, and be absolutely sure of your footing; a misstep can mean a nasty or possibly fatal fall.

- Standing dead trees and storm-damaged living trees can pose a real hazard to hikers and tent campers. These trees may have loose or broken limbs that could fall at any time. When choosing a spot to rest or a backcountry campsite, look up.

- Know the symptoms of hypothermia. Shivering and forgetfulness are the two most common indicators of this insipid killer. Hypothermia can occur at any elevation, even in the summer, especially when the hiker is wearing lightweight cotton clothing. If symptoms arise, get the victim shelter, hot liquids, and dry clothes or a dry sleeping bag.

- Take along your brain. A cool, calculating mind is the single most important piece of equipment you'll ever need on the trail. Think before you act. Watch your step. Plan ahead. Avoiding accidents before they happen is the best recipe for a rewarding and relaxing hike.

ANIMAL AND PLANT HAZARDS

TICKS

Ticks like to hang out in the brush that grows along trails. Hot summer months seem to explode their numbers, but you should be tick-aware during all months of the year. Ticks, which are arthropods and not insects, need a host to feast on in order to reproduce. The ticks that light onto you while you hike will be very small, sometimes so tiny that you won't be able to spot them. Primarily of two varieties, deer ticks and dog ticks, both need a few hours of actual attachment before they can transmit any disease they may harbor. Ticks may settle in shoes, socks, and hats and may take several hours to actually latch on. The best strategy is to visually check every half hour or so while hiking, do a thorough check before you get in the car, and then, when you take a posthike shower, do an even more thorough check of your entire body. Ticks that haven't attached are easily removed but not easily killed. If you pick off a tick in the woods, just toss it aside. If you find one on your body at home, dispatch it and then send it down the toilet. For ticks that have embedded, removal with tweezers is best.

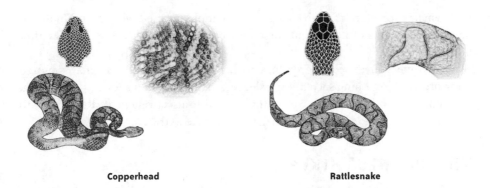

Copperhead   Rattlesnake

SNAKES

Tennessee is home to 32 types of snakes, 4 of which are venomous. Consider yourself lucky if you see a snake, acknowledging that snakes are part of the great Middle Tennessee ecosystem. Refrain from messing with them. All of the Volunteer State's venomous snakes have a vertical, elliptical-shaped pupil and are generally heavy bodied. The timber rattler and copperhead are found throughout Middle Tennessee. The two others, cottonmouth and pygmy rattler, can be found west of the Nashville Basin. You might spend a few minutes studying snakes before heading into the woods, but a good rule of thumb is to give whatever animal you encounter a wide berth and leave it alone.

POISON IVY, POISON OAK, POISON SUMAC

Recognizing poison ivy, oak, and sumac and avoiding contact with them is the most effective way to prevent the painful, itchy rashes associated with these plants. Poison ivy ranges from a thick tree-hugging vine to a shaded groundcover, three leaflets to a leaf; poison oak occurs as either a vine or shrub, with three leaflets as well; and poison sumac flourishes in swampland, each leaf containing 7 to 13 leaflets. Urushiol, the oil in the sap of these plants, is responsible for the rash. Usually within 12 to 14 hours of exposure (but sometimes much later), raised lines and/or blisters will appear, accompanied by a terrible itch. Refrain from scratching because bacteria under fingernails can cause infection and you will spread the rash to other parts of your body. Wash and dry the rash thoroughly, applying a calamine lotion or other product to help dry the rash. If itching or blistering is severe, seek medical attention. Remember that oil-contaminated clothes, pets, or hiking gear can easily cause an irritating rash on you or someone else, so wash not only any exposed parts of your body but also clothes, gear, and pets.

MOSQUITOES

Although it's very rare, individuals can become infected with the West Nile virus by being bitten by an infected mosquito. Culex mosquitoes, the primary varieties that can transmit West Nile virus to humans, thrive in urban rather than natural areas. They lay their eggs in stagnant water and can breed in any standing water that remains for more than five days. Most people infected with West Nile virus have no symptoms of illness, but some may become ill, usually 3 to 15 days after being bitten.

Anytime you expect mosquitoes to be buzzing around, you may want to wear protective clothing such as long sleeves, long pants, and socks. Loose-fitting, light-colored clothing is best. Spray clothing with insect repellent. Remember to follow the instructions on the repellent and to take extra care with children.

THE BUSINESS HIKER

Whether you're in the Nashville area on business as a resident or an out-of-towner, the hikes in this book afford the perfect opportunity to make a quick getaway from the demands of commerce. Some of the hikes classified as urban are located close to office areas and are easily accessible from downtown areas.

Instead of buying a burger down the street, pack a lunch and head for a nearby trail to take a relaxing break from the office or that tiresome convention. Or plan ahead and take along a small group of your business comrades. A well-planned half-day getaway is the perfect complement to a business stay in Nashville or any of the other close-in communities in the metropolitan area.

TRAIL ETIQUETTE

Whether you're on a city, county, state, or national park trail, always remember that great care and resources (from nature as well as from your tax dollars) have gone into creating these trails. Treat the trail, wildlife, and fellow hikers with respect. Here are a few general ideas to keep in mind while on the trail:

1. **Hike on open trails only. Respect trail and road closures (ask if you're not sure), avoid trespassing on private land, and obtain any required permits or authorization. Leave gates as you found them or as marked.**

2. **Leave no trace of your visit other than footprints. Be sensitive to the land beneath your feet. This also means staying on the trail and not creating any new trails. Be sure to pack out what you pack in. No one likes to see trash that someone else has left behind.**

3. **Never spook animals; give them extra room and time to adjust to you.**

4. **Plan ahead. Know your equipment, your ability, and the area in which you are hiking—and prepare accordingly. Be self-sufficient at all times; carry necessary supplies for changes in weather or other conditions. A well-executed trip is a satisfaction to you and not a burden or offense to others.**

5. **Be courteous to other hikers, bikers, and all people you meet while hiking.**

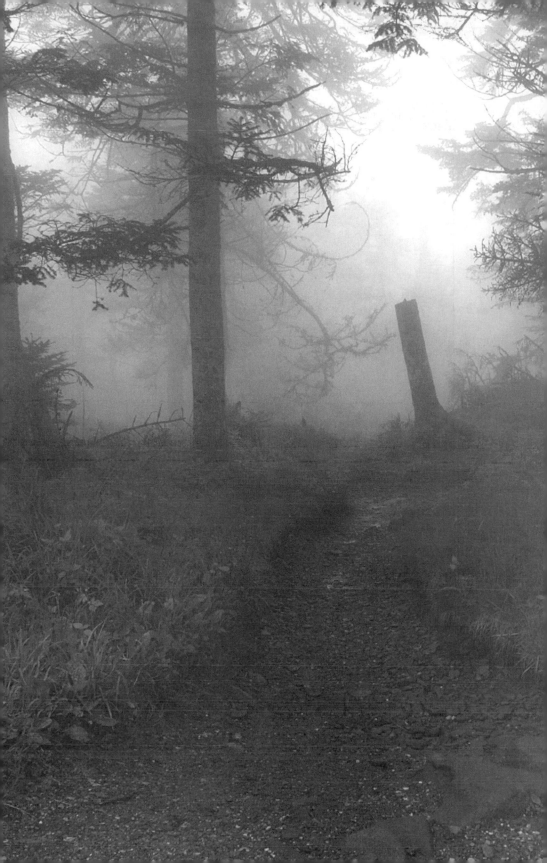

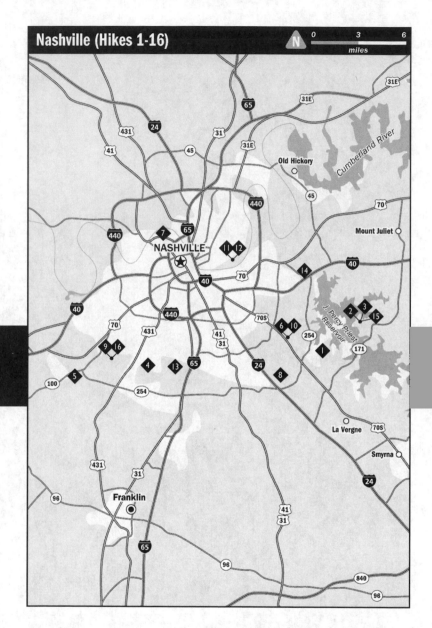

Nashville (Hikes 1-16)

N

0   3   6
miles

Old Hickory

Cumberland River

Mount Juliet

NASHVILLE

J. Percy Priest Reservoir

La Vergne

Smyrna

Franklin

1	Anderson Road Fitness Trail	14	
2	Bryant Grove Trail	18	
3	Couchville Lake Loop	22	
4	Ganier Ridge Loop	26	
5	Harpeth Woods Trail	29	
6	Lakeside Trail	32	
7	Metro Center Levee Greenway	35	
8	Mill Creek Greenway	38	
9	Mossy Ridge Trail	42	
10	Pinnacle Trail	46	
11	Shelby Bottoms Nature Park: East Loop	49	
12	Shelby Bottoms Nature Park: West Loop	53	
13	South Radnor Lake Loop	57	
14	Stones River Greenway of Nashville	61	
15	Volunteer–Day Loop	65	
16	Warner Woods Trail	69	

NASHVILLE

01 ANDERSON ROAD FITNESS TRAIL

KEY AT-A-GLANCE INFORMATION

LENGTH: 1.3 miles
CONFIGURATION: Loop
DIFFICULTY: Easy
SCENERY: Cedar forest, lakeshore
EXPOSURE: Mostly shady
TRAFFIC: Busy on nice-weather weekends and during summer
TRAIL SURFACE: Pavement, gravel
HIKING TIME: 1 hour
ACCESS: No fees to access trail, but fee for nearby recreation area
MAPS: Available on the Web at www.lrn.usace.army.mil/op/jpp/rec/arfitness.htm
FACILITIES: Restrooms, water at nearby picnic area

GPS Trailhead Coordinates

UTM Zone (WGS84)   16S
Easting   0535919
Northing   3995737
Latitude   N 36° 6' 26.3"
Longitude   W 86° 36' 3.3"

IN BRIEF

Part of the U.S. Army Corps of Engineers' Anderson Road Recreation Area, the Fitness Trail is a wooded oasis in the fast-growing area near Percy Priest Lake. Although labeled as a fitness trail, the path doesn't have exercise stations or any other man-made contraptions. It is an easy trail that wanders through cedar woods and glades, offering fantastic lake views as it skirts the shores of Percy Priest Lake.

DESCRIPTION

I would have named this Cedars by the Lake Trail, but I don't work for the Army Corps of Engineers, which dammed the Stones River to create Percy Priest Lake and developed several recreation areas on its shores. Name aside, the Fitness Trail makes for a quick and easy getaway for residents of the Music City. Most of the path skirts the shoreline, though the last portion turns away from the Priest Lake and heads toward a road that is part of the recreation area. You have to walk a bit of the road to complete the loop. Otherwise,

Directions

From Exit 219 on Interstate 40 east of downtown Nashville, take Stewarts Ferry Pike/Bell Road south 4.7 miles to Smith Springs Road. (Soon after leaving the Interstate, Stewarts Ferry Road becomes Bell Road.) Turn left on Smith Springs Road and follow it 1.1 miles to Anderson Road. Turn left on Anderson Road and follow it 1.3 miles. Turn left into the Fitness Trail parking area at the Couchville Pike intersection. The paved Fitness Trail starts at the back of the parking area toward the lake. Do not take the gravel path leading left from the parking area.

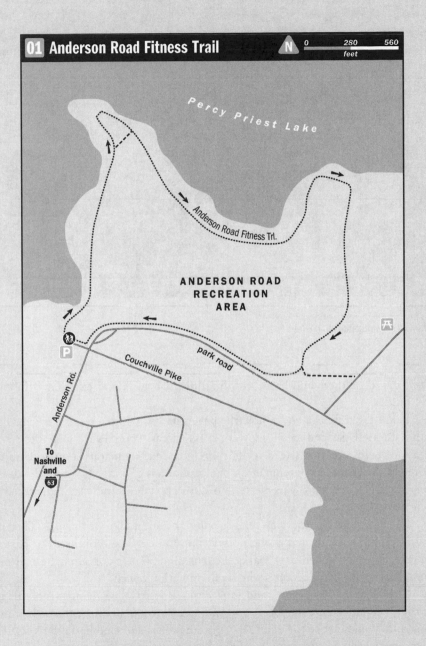

01 Anderson Road Fitness Trail

Percy Priest Lake

Anderson Road Fitness Trl.

ANDERSON ROAD
RECREATION
AREA

park road

Couchville Pike

Anderson Rd.

To
Nashville
and
63

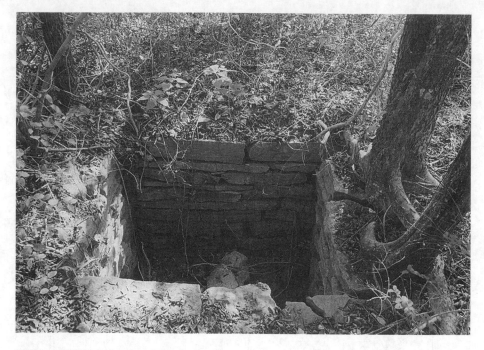

Old well from trailside homesite

hikers can do a there-and-back, avoiding the road walk and extending the hike to 2 miles.

Leave the trailhead and follow the paved pathway into a cedar forest broken with natural glades and small, mowed, grassy areas. Percy Priest Lake lies to the left, and many side paths lead to its shoreline. The main trail soon reaches the shores of the lake at a contemplation bench. Continue forward, noting the deciduous hackberry trees growing in the moister depressions and easily identified by their warty bark.

Reach a junction and stay left, curving around a lake peninsula. (The trail leading right shortcuts across the point.) The Fitness Trail continues to parallel the lakeshore; a wooden post marks the half-mile point. Soon after the half-mile point, reach the shoreline at another contemplation bench.

The seemingly low-slung and long Percy Priest Dam is easily visible to the north. Contemplate the numbers: The dam is 130 feet high, more than a half mile long, and 7 miles above the confluence of the Stones and Cumberland rivers. The reservoir drains 865 square miles of the Tennessee landscape; the primary drainages are the East Fork Stones and West Fork Stones rivers. Percy Priest Lake is 42 miles long and has 213 miles of curving shoreline and an average depth of 29 feet. This engineering project was initiated after World War II as part of the Flood Control Act of 1946. It was originally called Stewarts Ferry Reservoir but was changed to its current name to honor Tennessee Congressman J. Percy Priest. Dam construction began in 1963 and took five years. The purpose of the lake is to control flooding on the Cumberland River, generate hydropower, and provide public recreation.

Leave the dam vista, turn away from the lake, and soon look right for a short side trail. Just a few steps down this path are the remains of an old well. Back in settler days, a well was dug and abundant limestone rock was laid along the upper part of the hole to stabilize the well walls. Most of the old well has since been filled in, but you can still look down into it several feet. Thick cedar woods are slowly masking other remains of a homestead that was surely in the vicinity.

The Fitness Trail wanders through cedar glades and mixed deciduous woods. Scattered among the cedars is the black walnut. Middle Tennessee lies near the geographic center of the latter tree's range. The walnut, a hardwood with finely toothed compound leaves, is coveted so much for furniture that individual trees are sometimes stolen from private property. Since Colonial times, black walnuts have provided edible fare and a black dye made from their husks. Open up a walnut and your hands and clothes are sure to turn black from the dye. In fact, it is a rite of passage for children to ruin clothes from opening black walnuts. Squirrels and other wildlife avidly consume this nut.

The trail splits again. And a side trail leads left toward the picnic area. The Fitness Trail leads right and soon passes around vehicle-barrier boulders. At this point, hikers can backtrack 1.1 miles to the trailhead or take the recreation road leading right 0.2 miles, completing the loop at the trailhead.

NEARBY/RELATED ACTIVITIES

Anderson Recreation Area has a campground, a picnic area, a swim beach, and a boat ramp. For more information, call (615) 889-1975 or visit **www.orn.usace .army.mil/op/jpp/rec/arfitness.htm.**

02 BRYANT GROVE TRAIL

 KEY AT-A-GLANCE INFORMATION

LENGTH: 8 MILES

CONFIGURATION: There-and-back

DIFFICULTY: Moderate

SCENERY: Lake, cedar thickets, hardwood forest, cedar glades

EXPOSURE: More shady than sunny

TRAFFIC: Moderate

TRAIL SURFACE: Gravel, rocks, dirt

HIKING TIME: 4 hours

ACCESS: No fees or permits required

MAPS: Available on the Web at www.state.tn.us/environment/ parks/gis/pdf/printmaps/long hunter.pdf

FACILITIES: Restrooms, water at trailhead

SPECIAL COMMENTS: You can start trail on either end.

IN BRIEF

This there-and-back hike cruises through Long Hunter State Park, along the pretty shoreline of Percy Priest Lake. The walking is easy, but the total distance—if you make the entire hike—is 8 miles. You may see wading birds and waterfowl in season.

DESCRIPTION

The Bryant Grove Trail is your best bet for solitude at Long Hunter State Park. The path starts in the busy Couchville Lake Day Use Area and then heads east along the shore of Percy Priest Lake. The wide trail bed is easy to follow as it meanders through cedar thickets, oak–hickory forests, and cedar glades to swing around the Bryant Creek embayment. It ends at Bryant Grove Recreation Area, where picnic tables and a swim beach await. Be aware—this is not a loop trail. The 4 miles out, though easy with no real hills, require 4 miles back to the trailhead, unless you leave another car at Bryant Grove Recreation Area, which is a 7-mile drive from the Couchville Lake Area.

Start the Bryant Grove Trail by leaving the Couchville Lake Day Use Area and tracing the gravel path into cedar woods. Couchville

GPS Trailhead Coordinates

UTM Zone (WGS84) 16S

Easting 0541070

Northing 3994360

Latitude N 36° 5' 35.0"

Longitude W 86° 32' 37.5"

Directions

From Exit 226 on I-40 east of downtown Nashville, take South Mount Juliet Road, TN 171, south 4.2 miles. Veer right at the split as TN 171 becomes Hobson Pike. Continue forward 2.4 miles, turning left into the Couchville Day Use Area. Continue forward 0.4 miles and turn left into Area Two. Soon reach the parking area and trailhead. The trail starts near the playground on the right side of the parking area as you enter it.

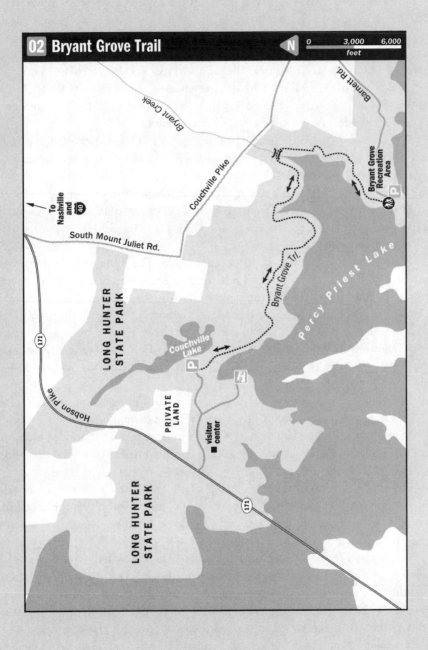

02 Bryant Grove Trail

N

0   3,000   6,000
feet

Barnett Rd.

Bryant Creek

Couchville Pike

Bryant Grove Recreation Area

To Nashville and 40

South Mount Juliet Rd.

Bryant Grove Trl.

Percy Priest Lake

LONG HUNTER STATE PARK

171

Couchville Lake

Hobson Pike

PRIVATE LAND

visitor center

171

LONG HUNTER STATE PARK

Lake and the Couchville Lake Trail are off to your left. Shortly pick up the old bed of O'Neals Ford Road. You'll notice that the canopy gives way overhead and Percy Priest Lake is off to your right. In the winter, when the lake pool is drawn down, you can see the rockiness of the lake bed. In the woods to your left, vast amounts of rock protrude above what little soil occurs in this karst topography, where the limestone lies at or near the land surface. Pockets of rich soil do occur here, which is usually indicated by the presence of oak–hickory forests. In less-rich soil, cedars dominate. The poorest soils or the areas with the least amount of dirt (and most exposed rock) will harbor cedar glades.

Wooden posts mark the trail's progression at half-mile increments. Climb a small hill just past the 0.5-mile post, then make a hard left, leaving the lake and roadbed. A sign here reads, "Trail Does Not Loop," reminding hikers that every step they hike out, they will have to hike back. Look for a crumbling, old stone wall in the woods off to your right. You may also see wooden posts supporting barbed wire. These lands, too rocky for large-scale agriculture, were used for grazing in prepark days.

Look left at the 1-mile post for a cedar glade. The Bryant Grove Trail veers right here and picks up another woods road to enter terrain that slopes toward the lake. Begin curving around the Bryant Creek embayment and arrive near the shore before reaching a signboard and kiosk indicating the halfway point of the trail at 2 miles. Just past the kiosk, the Bryant Grove Trail crosses an unnamed wet-weather stream. Rocks have been placed across the crossing, enabling hikers to keep their feet dry even after winter rains, when this stream is likely to be running. In fall, it may be nearly dry.

Keep curving around the cove, and soon you'll be traveling directly along the shoreline. Views stretch far onto Percy Priest Lake, and birds, such as herons, may be wading in the embayment. The Bryant Grove Trail continues along the shore to reach Bryant Creek at mile 2.8; a wooden bridge with handrails allows dry passage. Turn downstream along Bryant Creek, where you can see the stream flow into the lake. Look across the creek at a stone wall along the creek bank that kept Bryant Creek in check in days gone by. (The rich soil along the creek may have been used for a family's vegetable garden.) Another stone wall is visible across the water above the creek bank.

Pass a small feeder stream on a boardwalk, and look left for a larger glade growing up in young bushy cedars. The Bryant Grove Trail then enters a dense cedar thicket that forms a dark, cool pocket no matter the time of year. Emerge from the thicket and enter a gravelly glade at mile 3.4. The openness of the sky at this point will make you squint. This area contains the poorest of poor soil from a farmer's perspective but is rare, rich land to a botanist. Land isn't even the right word for this area because it really is an extensive flat of broken limestone rock. In the cracks and crevices are wildflowers and rare plants that grow only in these glades, making Middle Tennessee home to a unique environment in the United States.

Drift among more open glades, then ascend through a rocky hardwood forest to reach Bryant Grove Recreation Area at 4 miles. Here you'll find picnic tables, grills, a restroom, a boat launch, and a swim beach. If you haven't left a shuttle car here, it is time to backtrack to Couchville Lake Day Use Area.

Early to late spring is the best time to view wildflowers along this trail. However, keep in mind that heavy winter and spring rains tend to wash over the trail, rendering it impassable across Bryant Creek (despite the bridge) and over the O' Neals Ford roadbed from the Couchville Lake side. Call ahead if you are concerned about high water.

NEARBY/RELATED ACTIVITIES

The park has a fishing pier and rents canoes and small johnboats. No gas motors are allowed, which makes for a peaceful experience. For more information, call (615) 885-2422.

03 COUCHVILLE LAKE LOOP

KEY AT-A-GLANCE INFORMATION

LENGTH: 2 miles

CONFIGURATION: Loop

DIFFICULTY: Easy

SCENERY: Lakeside forest

EXPOSURE: Mostly shady

TRAFFIC: Busy on weekends and weekday afternoons

TRAIL SURFACE: Smooth asphalt

HIKING TIME: 1 hour

ACCESS: No fees or permits required

MAPS: Available on the Web at www.state.tn.us/environment/parks/gis/pdf/printmaps/long hunter.pdf

FACILITIES: Restrooms, water at trailhead

SPECIAL COMMENTS: This is a barrier-free trail. Couchville Lake is open to fishing. The state park has a fishing pier and rents canoes and small johnboats. No gas motors are allowed, which makes for a more peaceful experience. For more information call (615) 885-2422 or visit www.tnstateparks.com.

IN BRIEF

This easy trail circles Couchville Lake, which lies adjacent to Percy Priest Lake at Long Hunter State Park. The popular paved path winds through woods and has many side trails leading to small piers on the lake's edge. Tree- and plant-identification signs enhance the experience. And a 300-foot bridge that spans the lake offers panoramic views. You may also see wildlife on the lake and in the woods on quiet mornings.

DESCRIPTION

I think Long Hunter State Park did a fine job laying out this trail. The eight-foot-wide, nearly level path makes up in beauty what it lacks in challenge. But that is the very point of this trail—to be accessible for folks with disabilities as well as the average walker. Those developing Long Hunter State Park actually had no idea what a good recreation destination Couchville Lake would become because they had no idea Couchville Lake would ever exist. Before the Stones River was dammed and Percy Priest Lake was formed, the area that would later become Couchville Lake was just a big depression. When Percy Priest Lake filled, water seeped from the impoundment through underground passages to fill the

GPS Trailhead Coordinates

UTM Zone (WGS84) 16S

Easting   0541100

Northing   3994160

Latitude   N 36° 5' 34.4"

Longitude   W 86° 32' 37.1"

Directions

From Exit 226 on I-40 east of downtown Nashville, take South Mount Juliet Road, TN 171, south 4.2 miles. Veer right at the split as TN 171 becomes Hobson Pike. Continue forward 2.4 miles, turning left into the Couchville Day Use Area. Keep forward 0.4 miles and turn left into Area Two; soon you'll reach the parking area and trailhead. The trail starts near the fishing pier on the edge of Couchville Lake.

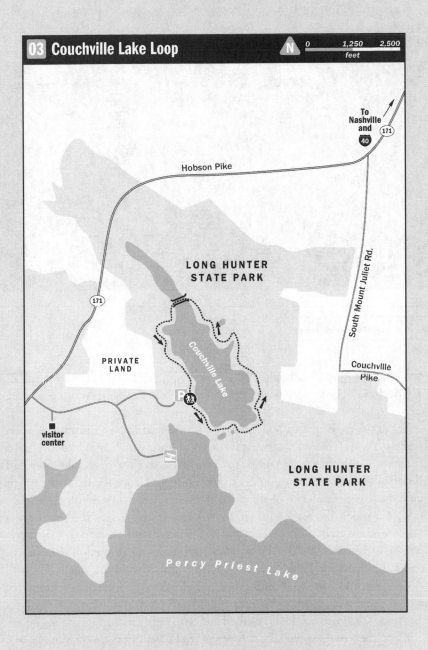

03 Couchville Lake Loop

N

0   1,250   2,500
feet

To
Nashville
and
40
171

Hobson Pike

171

LONG HUNTER
STATE PARK

South Mount Juliet Rd.

Couchville
Pike

PRIVATE
LAND

Couchville Lake

P

visitor
center

LONG HUNTER
STATE PARK

Percy Priest Lake

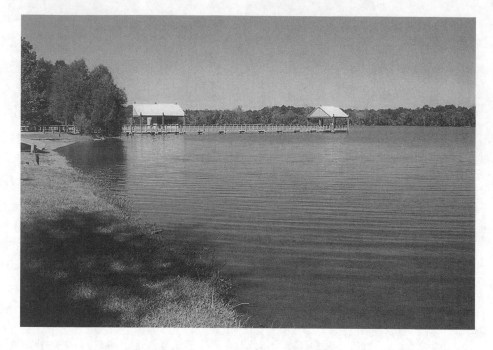

Pier stretches into Couchville Lake

depression, forming Couchville Lake. And this relationship between Percy Priest and Couchville continues: when Percy Priest Lake goes up or down, so goes Couchville Lake.

Leave the parking area and head toward the fishing pier and canoes stored at the lake's edge. Here you'll turn right onto the trail, which is marked in half-mile increments. Couchville Lake will be to your left. Leave the open lakeshore to find a woodland area of cedar, walnut, and oak. Soon you'll see the first of many interpretive signs, which inform hikers of the trees and plants around them.

At 0.2 miles, the level path circles to the left and passes the first of several small lakeside observation piers. Bird boxes are perched on poles in the lake. Soon you'll pass a sinkhole/pond on your right that was formed in the same manner as was Couchville Lake. A smaller pond is just beyond the first.

Circle around the lake and enter a cedar grove. The cedar, which often grows in poor soils, is important for wildlife. Birds use its thin, stringy bark to build nests, songbirds eat its berrylike fruit, and deer feed on its green foliage.

More piers jut into the lake before the trail passes over a dry drainage at mile 1. Ahead are resting benches covered by a shelter that would come in handy during a summer thunderstorm. Look for a willow-rimmed pond to your right, noting that the land bridge between Couchville Lake and the pond is very narrow. These are black willows, the most common of a dozen willows that grow in North America. These trees grow in wet soils along rivers and lakes, acting as a

natural erosion barrier. In pioneer days, willow charcoal was a source of gunpow-
der; nowadays, it is used in furniture, baskets, barrels, and pulpwood. In Middle
Tennessee, willow rarely grows to commercial-timber size as it does in the lower
Mississippi River Valley.

At mile 1.4, span Couchville Lake on a 300-foot wooden bridge that offers
the best lake vistas on the entire trail. Imagine the scene before you as a wooded
depression, like it was before Percy Priest Lake dam was built. Persimmon trees
grow beyond the bridge; look for furrowed bark broken in squares. In the fall,
you will see sweet orange persimmon fruit among the leaves and overhead, still
on the tree even after its leaves have fallen. This fruit recalls the flavor of dates.
Hard, unripe persimmons are unpalatable, though, so make sure to get a softer,
riper fruit. In fact, many old-timers believe persimmons shouldn't be eaten until
after the first frost. Native Americans made persimmon bread and also stored the
dried fruit like prunes. Possums, raccoons, skunks, deer, and birds enjoy the fruit,
which contains a few seeds. I love persimmons too.

The trail curves around a low drainage to the right, where hackberries grow
in a nearly pure stand. These trees, which have gray bark dotted with obvious
corky warts, favor moist soils such as this drainage. The trail treads farther from
the lake, and dirt paths reach out to more small docks that extend into the water.
Just ahead you will find the fishing pier, a picnic area, boat-rental headquarters,
and the end of the loop.

04 GANIER RIDGE LOOP

**KEY AT-A-GLANCE
INFORMATION**

LENGTH: 2.4 miles
CONFIGURATION: Loop
DIFFICULTY: Moderate
SCENERY: Wooded hills and valleys
EXPOSURE: Shady
TRAFFIC: Fairly busy
TRAIL SURFACE: Dirt, rocks
HIKING TIME: 1.8 hours
ACCESS: No fees or permits required
MAPS: Available on the Web at
www.state.tn.us/environment/
parks/RadnorLake
FACILITIES: Water spigot, restrooms
at trailhead

IN BRIEF

This loop explores the high and the low of
Radnor Lake State Natural Area. Depart from
the less-used east side of the park, then climb
steeply up the Ganier Ridge Trail into the highest hills in Nashville. Just as you get accustomed
to the oak forest up there, the loop drops down
to a rich hollow and reaches the north shore of
Radnor Lake, a haven for waterfowl. Finish
your hike in the flat alongside Radnor Lake.

DESCRIPTION

This hike climbs to about as high as you can
get in the Nashville Basin. The areas around it
were once simple farms, and the rugged hills
have been logged over. But the story of Radnor Lake begins when the Louisville and Nashville Railroad, or L&N, purchased this parcel
of land. Back in 1919, the railroad impounded
Otter Creek to create Radnor Lake and used
its water for steam engines at the adjacent
Radnor Yards. The land around the lake was
used as a hunting preserve for the elite at
L&N. These officials soon recognized the
heavy use of the lake by native and migratory
birds and declared the area a wildlife sanctuary at the urging of the Tennessee Ornithological Society. Ganier Ridge is named after

GPS Trailhead
Coordinates

UTM Zone (WGS84) 16S
Easting 0518460
Northing 3990210
Latitude N 36° 3' 28.9"
Longitude W 86° 47' 43.1"

Directions

From Exit 78 on I-65 south of downtown Nashville, take Harding Place Road 0.4 miles west
to intersect US 31, Franklin Pike. Turn left on
Franklin Pike and follow it 1.3 miles south to
Otter Creek Road. Turn right on Otter Creek
Road and follow it 1.2 miles to the parking
area on your right. The Access Trail starts
beside the parking permit–restroom building
at the top of the parking area.

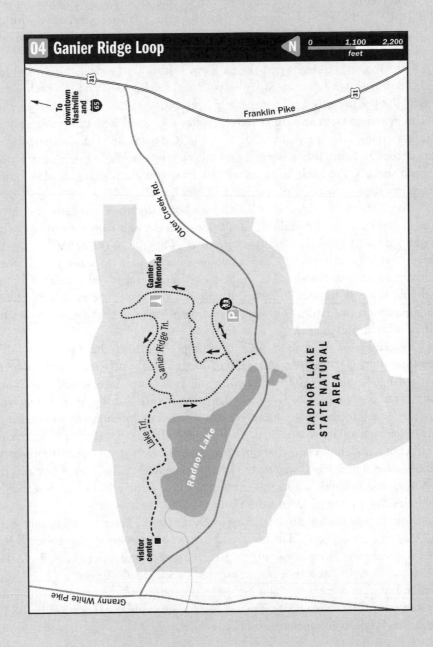

04 Ganier Ridge Loop

N

0   1,100   2,200
feet

Albert Ganier, an active member of the society that swayed the L&N to preserve the area. To this day, hikers of this loop can see the small plaque commemorating him. In 1973, the state of Tennessee purchased the 1,060-acre preserve with the help of citizen donations. The preserve remains an oasis of nature in the middle of Nashville.

The Access Trail leads past the park pay station into a viney hardwood forest. Climb west with Ganier Ridge to your right. Then descend to reach a trail junction at 0.2 miles. Turn right, passing over a dry branch on a footbridge, then ascend by switchbacks up Ganier Ridge. Notice the wire fence; this was part of an old farm, one of the early incarnations of the Radnor Lake area. Ganier Ridge is part of the Overton Hills, named for John Overton, one of Nashville's early movers and shakers. He likely once owned the land you are walking on. His home, Travellers Rest, is just east of here off of Franklin Pike.

Top out on the ridge in a hickory-and-oak–dominated forest. Stay at or near the ridgeline. The walking is glorious among the sometimes-windswept hardwoods atop this hill. Swing around to the left side of the actual high point before reaching mile 1 and a contemplation bench that faces the plaque commemorating Albert Ganier. The stone-based memorial is only about two feet high and is easily missed. In fact, if it weren't for Ganier we may have missed out entirely on this park. The slight rumbling of autos in the distance belies the wild aura that pulses here.

Descend from the plaque, then turn sharply left down the now-rocky ridge. The forest here is more open and stunted, due to the south-facing rocky soil being parched by the sun. This contrasts with the rich cove—into which the Ganier Ridge Trail descends by steps—where hardwoods such as tulip, maple, and sycamore grow tall in the thick, moist soil. Soon, cross an intermittent streamed by bridge to reach an old woods road. The Ganier Ridge Trail turns left here, tracing a carpet of woodchips over what once may have been a logging road. Intersect the Lake Trail at mile 1.7 and stay on the left, keeping Radnor Lake to your right; the impoundment is visible through the trees. The land flattens but is still bisected by small drainages coming down from Ganier Ridge.

You'll cross a substantial drainage by footbridge. Then the trail briefly splits and merges back together. The high road passes by a contemplation bench, while the low road stays along the drainage. Reach another trail junction. And stay left again, as the right-hand trail leads to Otter Creek Road. Ascend a rib ridge of Ganier Ridge and meet yet another junction, one you are familiar with—the beginning of the Ganier Ridge Trail. Keep forward and backtrack 0.2 miles on the Access Trail to complete the loop.

NEARBY/RELATED ACTIVITIES

The busier west side of the park has a nature center. They have an excellent slide show available upon request, as well as other nature displays. For more information, call (615) 373-3467 or visit **www.tnstateparks.com**.

HARPETH WOODS TRAIL 05

IN BRIEF

Part of the Warner Parks trail system, this hike combines human and natural history as it loops through the Harpeth Hills, a collection of ridges southwest of downtown Nashville. First, the Harpeth Woods Trail follows a portion of the old Natchez Trace before visiting a long-abandoned rock quarry in the Little Harpeth River Valley. It then climbs a knob, passing some old-growth trees before descending back along a small stream to once again pick up the old trace.

DESCRIPTION

This loop makes a great hike for those who don't want to spend an entire day driving to and from the trailhead. Moreover, it offers an escape into the forest and a day's worth of exercise.

First, stop at the covered trailside kiosk near the parking area. Turn right and follow the blue blazes southwesterly down the straight dirt-and-rock path, which is a remnant of the original Natchez Trace before it was rerouted farther south. This more-than-two-centuries-old trail was considered the "interstate" of travel between Natchez, Mississippi, and Nashville in the early 1800s.

Continuing, you'll span Vaughns Creek on a footbridge. You may walk around the

KEY AT-A-GLANCE INFORMATION

LENGTH: 2.5 miles
CONFIGURATION: Loop
DIFFICULTY: Easy
SCENERY: Hardwood and cedar forest, small creek
EXPOSURE: Mostly shady
TRAFFIC: Busy on weekends
TRAIL SURFACE: Dirt, rocks
HIKING TIME: 1.3 hours
ACCESS: No fees or permits
MAPS: Available on the Web at www.nashville.gov/parks/images/previous/edwinwarner_map.jpg
FACILITIES: Restrooms, water at nature center
SPECIAL COMMENTS: Add Owl Hollow Trail for a 2.8-mile loop.

Directions ⟶

From Exit 199 on I-40 west of downtown Nashville, take Old Hickory Boulevard 4 miles south to intersect TN 100. Turn left on TN 100 and follow it 0.3 miles to the Edwin Warner Park trailhead, which will be on your right. Turn right, and then park in the trailhead parking to the right. The blue-blazed path starts near the trail kiosk.

GPS Trailhead Coordinates

UTM Zone (WGS84) 16S
Easting 0508120
Northing 3990260
Latitude N 36° 3' 32.5"
Longitude W 86° 54' 36.3"

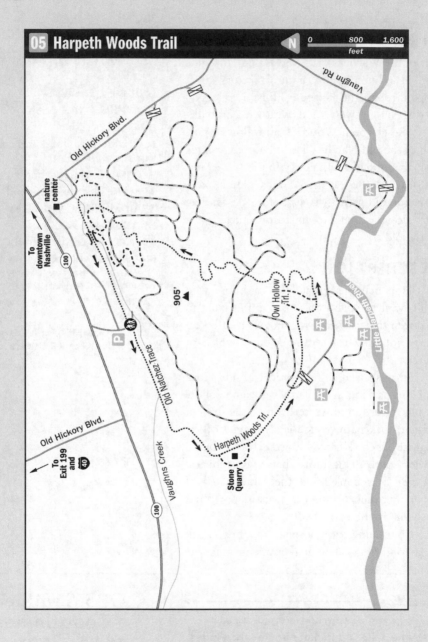

05 **Harpeth Woods Trail**

N

0   800   1,600
feet

bridge, as Vaughns Creek is most often low or dry at this point. Then keep forward in deep woods, only to leave the old trace and climb a rocky hillside to meet a side trail. Take this short trail to the quarry, where the open brightness offers great contrast to the shadier woods. Stone was first extracted here by settlers of the Little Harpeth River Valley and later by Great Depression–era workers for the gates and walls you see around the park.

Return to the main trail to bisect a closed paved road, and you'll arrive at a forest heavy with cedar trees. Many of these are large for cedars but don't get much acclaim because the large cedars aren't nearly as large as the huge oaks you will eventually pass. The tree canopy breaks open as the Harpeth Woods Trail meets the Owl Hollow Trail at mile 1.3. This interpretive trail (get an informative booklet about it at the park nature center) circles the valley to your left.

The Harpeth Woods Trail continues forward to reach a picnic shelter, near the Little Harpeth River, before ascending a knob via switchbacks that pass the other end of the Owl Hollow Trail along the way. The trail nearly runs into the aforementioned huge oak tree, complete with ferns growing in a crook on the lower limbs. These are known as resurrection ferns, as they curl up when the weather is dry, then unfurl and become green after rains; they are more common farther south, especially in Florida.

Leave the ferns behind, cross another paved road (most of Edwin Warner Park's paved roads, once used as scenic drives, are closed to autos and traveled by hikers and bikers), and keep switchbacking upward to reach the crest of the knob. Work around the knob, which reaches over 900 feet in elevation and stands nearly 300 feet above Vaughns Creek. And stay with the blue blazes, as the Harpeth Woods Trail switchbacks downhill to meet the Nature Trail, then bisects another closed paved road. You'll approach a huge beech tree beside an intermittent streambed before meeting the old Natchez Trace once again at a trail junction; the path that runs forward will lead you to the nature center. Turn left on the trace and follow the trail to a bridge over Vaughns Creek. At this point Vaughns Creek runs perennially, unlike farther downstream where it simply dries up at the surface in late summer and fall. Keep forward on the old trace with the knob to your left and a field to your right to shortly complete the loop.

NEARBY/RELATED ACTIVITIES

The Warner Parks Nature Center is a point of pride for the Nashville park system. It offers wide-ranging environmental education programs for visitors of all ages. Its large learning center has an exhibit hall, outdoor classroom, and more. Also in the area are a library with a large collection of natural-history books, a teaching pond, and a wildflower garden. For more information, call (615) 352-6299 or visit **www.nashville.gov/parks/wpnc**.

06 LAKESIDE TRAIL

KEY AT-A-GLANCE INFORMATION

LENGTH: 2 miles
CONFIGURATION: Loop
DIFFICULTY: Easy
SCENERY: Rock-strewn forest
EXPOSURE: Shady
TRAFFIC: Busy on weekends
TRAIL SURFACE: Dirt, rocks
HIKING TIME: 1 hour
ACCESS: No fees or permits
MAPS: Hamilton Creek Trails, available online at www.lrn.usace.army.mil/op/jpp/rec/hamilton.htm
FACILITIES: Restrooms, water at parking area

IN BRIEF

This trail makes a loop on U.S. Army Corps of Engineers land. The terrain in this area has some vertical variation in the oak-and-cedar forest through which it travels. The trail makes for a good leg stretcher near Percy Priest Lake.

DESCRIPTION

Lakeside Trail makes an elongated loop near the shores of Percy Priest Lake, traveling beside the lake but not going along the shore of the impoundment. Originally designed for mountain bikers, this path is open to hikers and is also used regularly by walkers and bikers. Consider doing this trail during off times, such as early morning or on weekdays, because on dry weekends there'll be too many mountain bikers on the path for you to have a pleasurable experience. When the trail is muddy, however, bikers are encouraged to stay off the trail.

This trail puts walkers on the slower but surer way to fitness. Even though many folks think walking is too easy to be of great health benefit, if done on a regular schedule it can lower your resting heart rate, reduce your blood pressure, increase the efficiency of your

GPS Trailhead Coordinates

UTM Zone (WGS84) 16S
Easting   0533720
Northing 3995490
Latitude N 36° 6' 17.9"
Longitude W 86° 37' 31.2"

Directions

From Exit 219 on I-40 east of downtown Nashville, take Stewarts Ferry Pike south. Soon after leaving the Interstate, Stewarts Ferry Road becomes Bell Road. Keep forward a total of 3.1 miles from I-40. Turn left on Hamilton Creek Road and follow it just a short distance. Then take the first right, heading downhill to a large parking area. The Lakeside Trail starts in the right corner of the parking area as you are driving in.

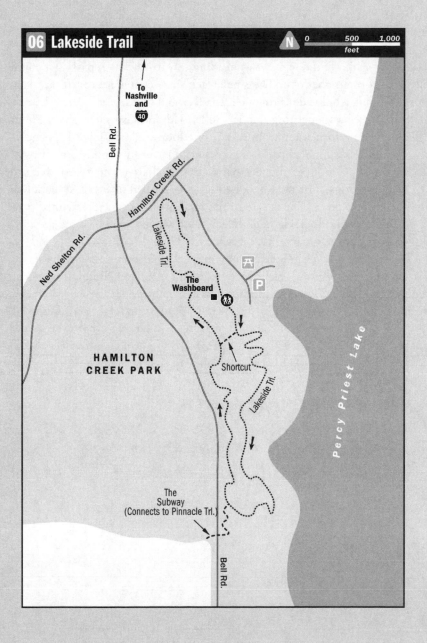

06 Lakeside Trail

N

0   500   1,000
feet

To
Nashville
and
40

Bell Rd.

Hamilton Creek Rd.

Ned Shelton Rd.

Lakeside Trl.

The
Washboard

P

Shortcut

Lakeside Trl.

HAMILTON
CREEK PARK

Percy Priest Lake

The
Subway
(Connects to Pinnacle Trl.)

Bell Rd.

heart and lungs, and help you burn excess calories. Moreover, it has the lowest dropout rate of any form of exercise.

Start this walk by leaving the parking area and immediately spanning a streambed on a low bridge. The path travels through a cedar coppice, then reaches a trail junction, which is the beginning of the loop. Turn left and begin working over hills and down swales heading toward the lake, passing a connector trail that shortcuts the loop. The singletrack path comes nearest to the lake just before climbing a hill and nearing Bell Road. At 0.8 miles, you'll reach the Subway, a path that uses a tunnel to go under Bell Road and also intersects the Pinnacle Trail (for more information about this 5-mile loop trail, see Hike 10, page 46).

The Lakeside Trail dips to cross some boardwalks in an area heavy with reindeer moss. Continue, roughly paralleling Bell Road, in forest that's dense with rock outcrops. The area may be better described as a limestone landscape over which trees grow. The nature of the land is evident in such named places as the Washboard and Rock Garden, the latter of which is met by the Lakeside Trail just before it begins to curve back toward the lake.

Pass through alternating hardwood and cedar forests, crossing the small flow of Twin Springs. Springs are important in this dry land. Rainfall is more than adequate in Middle Tennessee, so it is not the problem—it's what happens to the rain after it falls. With much of the water running underground due to all the sinks, it's no surprise that this dribble of water, which might not even be noticed in other parts of the state, is named here. Here the trail soon reaches the end of the loop. Turn left and walk a short distance to the trailhead.

NEARBY/RELATED ACTIVITIES

Hamilton Creek Park has picnic areas, lake access, BMX biking, and mountain biking. For more information, call (615) 862-8472.

METRO CENTER LEVEE GREENWAY

IN BRIEF

This elevated greenway travels atop a U.S. Army Corps of Engineers–built levee and provides a pleasant venue near downtown Nashville. Don't let its urban setting deter you from checking it out.

DESCRIPTION

I admit to being skeptical before trying this trail. However, after doing it, I give it a ringing endorsement. This 3-mile one-way path is being connected to downtown Nashville, which will expand the greenway system of the metro area. The story of this greenway begins in the early 1970s when the U.S. Army Corps of Engineers built a levee to protect the flats beside the river here, so businesses could develop. In the 1990s, the Corps determined the levee needed to be raised to meet new flood-control standards. The city and the Corps worked together to develop this trail along the improved levee. After a cost of $7.5 million, the trail was completed and opened for use in July 2003. Walkers, runners, and bicyclists all enjoy this path. Many employees of adjacent businesses utilize the trail at lunchtime.

The well-manicured trailhead serves greenway users heading along the Metro

KEY AT-A-GLANCE INFORMATION

LENGTH: 5.8 miles there and back
CONFIGURATION: Linear
DIFFICULTY: Moderate due to distance
SCENERY: Cumberland River, businesses and offices
EXPOSURE: Mostly sunny
TRAFFIC: Moderate
TRAIL SURFACE: Asphalt
HIKING TIME: 2.5 hours
ACCESS: No fees or permits
MAPS: Available on the Web at www.nashville.gov/greenways
FACILITIES: None

Directions

From Exit 85 (Rosa Parks Boulevard, State Capital, US 41A) on I-65 near downtown, take US 41A north toward Metro Center. Follow Rosa L. Parks/US 41A north for 0.4 miles to Vantage Way. Turn right on Vantage Way and follow it 0.5 miles. Turn right on Great Circle Road and follow it 0.3 miles to dead end at the trailhead, near the I-65 overpass spanning the Cumberland River.

GPS Trailhead Coordinates

UTM Zone (WGS 84) 16S
Easting   0519310
Northing   4005290
Latitude   N 36° 11' 32.2"
Longitude   W 86° 47' 7.0"

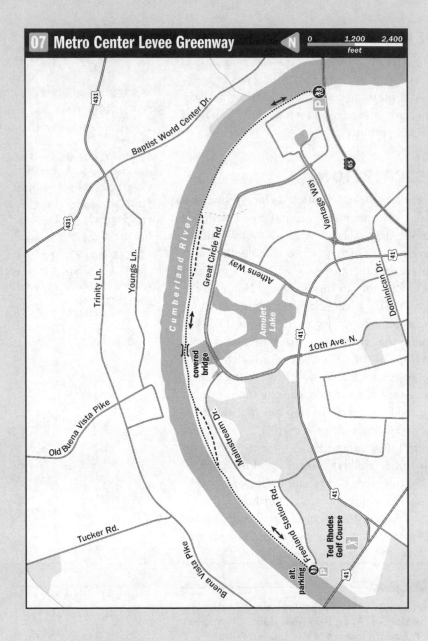

07 Metro Center Levee Greenway

Center Levee and the greenway heading into downtown Nashville. This trek heads toward the river, then joins the levee as it goes away from I-65. The paved trail is about 8 feet wide and roughly parallels the shoreline of the Cumberland River. Interesting shaded rest stops incorporate aquatic art reflecting the water. Art is also integrated into the concrete floodwall, the decorative trailside fences, and even the pavement!

Travel the path resting atop a berm straddling the margin between businesses to your left and the Cumberland River to your right. Make no mistake— this isn't a wilderness hike, but it is a not-to-be-overlooked exercise venue. Think of it as a way of varying your outdoor experiences. Be prepared for open conditions, as shade is short. Brush, riprap, and some trees—hackberry and sycamore— extend toward the river. Cottonwoods are also prevalent. The far shoreline is populated with occasional houses and businesses atop bluffs and hills.

At 0.9 miles, the levee splits, and you have a trail that runs closer to the river. Take this lower path, which soon rejoins the main levee trail. At 1.5 miles, you'll arrive at a "new-fashioned covered bridge." The 150-foot cylindrical screen tunnel through which you pass actually serves to hide a water-pumping station. This is also part of the integrated functional art found along the greenway. Landward views here include Amulet Lake.

At 1.8 miles, the trail splits again. Take the route that descends toward the river to enjoy the only shady section of trail. The paths rejoin at 2.2 miles, and you're once again atop the levee. The trail now curves southwesterly and soon reaches the Freeland Station Road trailhead at 2.9 miles. In case you want to just go one way and use a shuttle from the Great Circle Road trailhead, take Great Circle Road to Mainstream Drive. Turn right on Mainstream Drive, then take another right onto Freeland Station Road and follow it to dead end at this western trailhead.

NEARBY/RELATED ACTIVITIES

Stay tuned, as you will be able to use the Great Circle Road trailhead to access downtown Nashville via a greenway connecting to the already-built portions of Downtown Greenway in the heart of Music City.

08 MILL CREEK GREENWAY

KEY AT-A-GLANCE INFORMATION

LENGTH: 2.6 miles

CONFIGURATION: Loop plus there-and-back

DIFFICULTY: Easy

SCENERY: Urban interface, streamside woods

EXPOSURE: More sun than shade

TRAFFIC: Moderate to heavy on weekends

TRAIL SURFACE: Paved

HIKING TIME: 1.75 hours

ACCESS: No fees or permits

MAPS: Printable map at www.nashville.gov/greenways

FACILITIES: Restrooms at Antioch Community Center

IN BRIEF

This greenway is an urban classic, tucked away in a heavily developed area of Antioch adjacent to Interstate 24. It uses not only lands along the surprisingly pretty Mill Creek but also public property on the edge of Antioch Middle School and Antioch Community Center.

DESCRIPTION

Mill Creek is doing its best to remain a beautiful stream. In fact, the water coloration is still bluish, and paddlers can be found plying Mill Creek in spring and early summer. You arrived here on Blue Hole Road, named for a deep spot in the creek that has an especially deep-blue cast. A canoe-manufacturing company, Blue Hole Canoe, was named after this stream.

This walk begins on Whittmore Branch, a feeder stream of Mill Creek. Whittmore Branch is located behind the trailhead kiosk. From here, turn left and head upstream, with the creek to your right and Antioch Community Center to your left; I-24 is noisily close.

The greenway begins circling around the community center to pass under Blue Hole Road. A field and play area are located adjacent to the community center. The trail then squeezes behind Antioch Middle School, which longtime Antioch residents recall was

GPS Trailhead Coordinates

UTM Zone (WGS84) 16S

Easting 0529423

Northing 3990160

Latitude N 36° 3' 26.4"

Longitude W 86° 40' 24.2"

Directions

From Exit 59, Bell Road, on I-24 southeast of downtown Nashville, take Bell Road west 0.8 miles to Blue Hole Road. Turn right on Blue Hole Road and follow it 7 miles to reach the Antioch Community Center. The greenway starts at the back of the parking area.

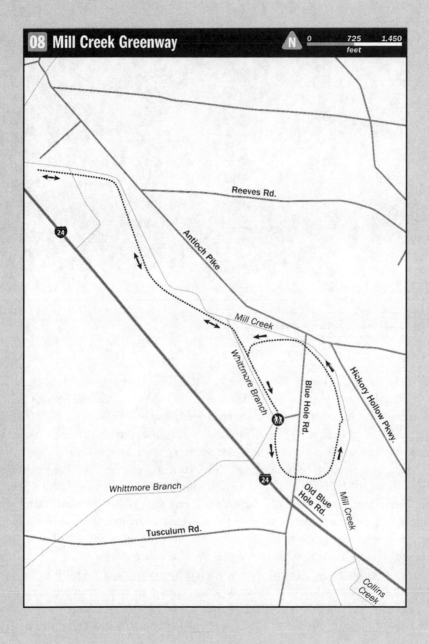

08 Mill Creek Greenway

N

0   725   1,450
feet

Reeves Rd.

24

Antioch Pike

Mill Creek

Whittmore Branch

Blue Hole Rd.

Hickory Hollow Pkwy.

24

Whittmore Branch

Old Blue Hole Rd.

Mill Creek

Tusculum Rd.

Collins Creek

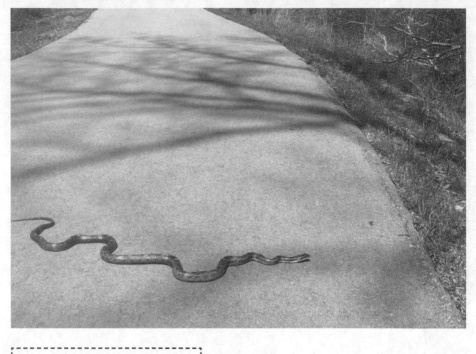

Even snakes use the Mill Creek Greenway.

once the Antioch High School. Soon you'll saddle alongside Mill Creek to your right. Look over the creek's still-bluish cast. At 0.6 miles, the trail passes beneath Blue Hole Road again, this time under a bridge spanning Mill Creek. When the creek floods, this part of the greenway can become muddy, though the trail is scraped clean by the city as soon as the water recedes.

The greenway continues along Mill Creek to complete the loop portion of the walk at 0.8 miles. Turn right, continuing downstream along Mill Creek. In days long past, early Nashvillians set up a gristmill on this stream, using water power to grind corn into meal, giving the stream its name. The greenway spans a feeder stream on a sturdy iron bridge, then climbs a bit of a hill as it works around a bluff. This segment of the greenway is more shaded.

Even though this greenway is bordered by civilization on both sides, it still offers refuge for wildlife, even snakes, as shown in the accompanying photo. Greenways such as this one, situated along a stream, protect wetlands and help with flood control, thanks to preserved and nonchannelized streams that absorb excess runoff. Continue downstream and enjoy the scenery as you pass a second bridge at 1.5 miles; the stream traveling underneath also feeds Mill Creek. Just ahead, at 1.6 miles, the Mill Creek Greenway currently ends. It is 1 mile back to the trailhead.

Keep apprised, as this greenway will be extended. Plans are underway to extend the paved path along Mill Creek to a trailhead on Richards Road, then onward to Ezell Park on Harding Place Road. A portion of the greenway in Ezell Park is already completed.

Greenways such as this provide community benefits, and you will see many people exercising along the path. And as Nashville's greenway system becomes more extended and connected, its paths will be used as transportation corridors.

NEARBY/RELATED ACTIVITIES

The trailhead is located at the Antioch Community Center, which holds classes and programs for kids and adults. To see what is going on there, please call the community center at (615) 315-9363.

09 MOSSY RIDGE TRAIL

KEY AT-A-GLANCE INFORMATION

LENGTH: 4.5 miles

CONFIGURATION: Loop

DIFFICULTY: Moderate

SCENERY: Woodlands

EXPOSURE: Nearly all shady

TRAFFIC: Moderate on weekends, some noise from TN 100

TRAIL SURFACE: Dirt, some rocks

HIKING TIME: 2.3 hours

ACCESS: No fees or permits

MAPS: Available on the Web at www.nashville.gov/parks/images/previous/percywarner_map.gif

FACILITIES: Portable restroom at Deep Well trailhead

IN BRIEF

The Mossy Ridge Trail is the longest of the three loop footpaths in the Warner Parks. It is the quietest and least used loop as well. An ideal training hike, the path leaves the Deep Well trailhead and winds through rich hollows and dry ridges of the Harpeth Hills, making frequent but never sustained elevation changes. Scattered in the woods are big trees and a spring-fed waterfall.

DESCRIPTION

At 4.5 miles, the Mossy Ridge Trail qualifies as a full-fledged hike that will not disappoint. If it weren't for some park road crossings and a little noise from TN 100, hikers would think they were in a remote swath of Middle Tennessee back in the days when Nashvillians traveled by horse. You will be traveling by foot in cove hardwood forests and along hickory–oak–cedar ridges in Percy Warner Park, where the hiking rivals any city park in the country.

Leave the covered trailside kiosk and trace the red blazes forward to a trail junction, crossing the wide, yellow-blazed Old Beech Bridle Path for the first of many times. The Warner Woods Trail goes off to the left, and the Mossy Ridge Trail goes to the right, swinging

GPS Trailhead Coordinates

UTM Zone (WGS84) 16S

Easting   0511030

Northing   3992340

Latitude   N 36° 4' 42.2"

Longitude   W 86° 52' 47.4"

Directions

From the point where TN 100 begins at US 70 near the Belle Meade Post Office, head west on TN 100 1.7 miles to the large stone gates on the left that mark the Deep Well entrance of Percy Warner Park. Turn left from TN 100 and pass through the gates, staying right when the road splits. Reach the Deep Well trailhead parking at 0.6 miles. The Mossy Ridge Trail starts behind the trailside kiosk.

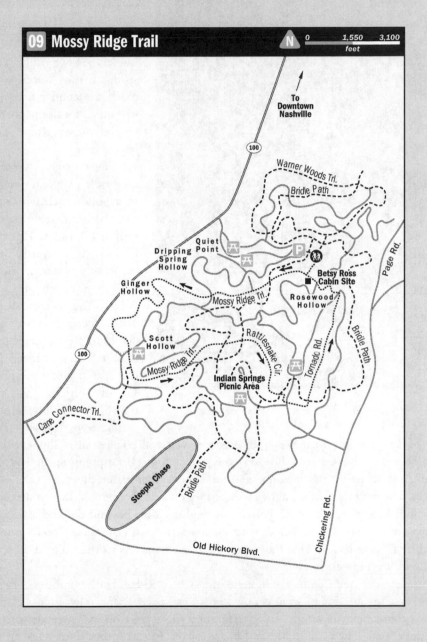

09 Mossy Ridge Trail

N

0   1,550   3,100
feet

To
Downtown
Nashville

100

Warner Woods Trl.

Bridle Path

Page Rd.

Quiet
Point

Dripping
Spring
Hollow

P

Betsy Ross
Cabin Site

Ginger
Hollow

Mossy Ridge Trl.

Rosewood
Hollow

Scott
Hollow

Rattlesnake Cir.

Mossy Ridge Trl.

Tornado Rd.

Bridle Path

100

Indian Springs
Picnic Area

Cane Connector Trl.

Steeple Chase

Bridle Path

Chickering Rd.

Old Hickory Blvd.

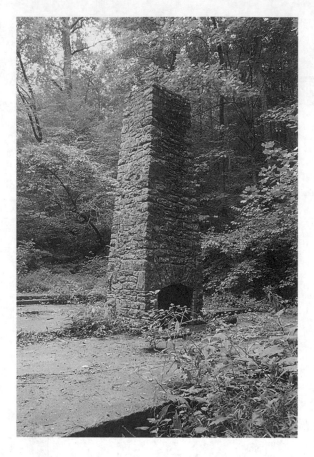

Chimney from the
Betsy Ross cabin

alongside a hillside out-cropped with mossy rocks. Look to your right at a spring below. Soon you'll reach a second junction at 0.1 mile; the loop portion of the Mossy Ridge Trail begins here.

Turn right, crossing the bridle path and descend to a hollow rich with tulip trees before reaching a side trail at 0.5 miles. This trail leads right 70 yards on a surprisingly narrow ridge-line to a bench at Quiet Point. The Mossy Ridge Trail keeps forward and climbs to meet a scenic park road on Gum Ridge. The path drops along the north side of the ridge into Drip-ping Spring Hollow. Here a spring seep drops over an exposed rock line to make a wet-weather waterfall. The trail is slippery as it bridges the exposed rock line, so consider taking the Dripping Spring Bypass, which skirts below the rock line and the wet-weather waterfall to meet the main trail. The path then winds above Ginger Hollow and Dome Hollow and descends by long switchbacks to near TN 100. A field is visible beyond the line of woods. Cross another park road before reaching a junction with the Cane Creek Connec-tor Trail at mile 1.9. This trail leads right and connects to the trails at adjacent Edwin Warner Park.

The ups and downs continue as the Mossy Ridge Trail continues forward and ascends the side of what is now known as Mossy Ridge, where moss carpets the ground below scattered oaks, cedar, and rocks. Stay on the ridgeline to cross a park road. Then follow the red blazes of the footpath, but don't pick up the horse trail, which also crosses the road. Soon cross the bridle path twice in suc-cession and ascend to a hilltop known as Rattlesnake Circle. Make easy tracks among both spindly and large trees. Drop down to near the Indian Springs Picnic Area. Reach a paved road and turn left on the paved road, bridging a streambed.

Cross a road and a mowed field before reentering forestland. Make a long switch-back, working up to the ridgeline known as Tornado Road, where the trailside is adorned with the first tree-identification signs. The walking is easy here. The next ridgeline over to the east is visible. And Tornado Road ends all too soon as it drops to a paved park road. Turn left, following the paved park road, veer right, and drop into Basswood Hollow.

Middle Tennessee is near the southern end of the basswood's growth range. This tree's roundish leaves are almost as wide as they are long, and its bark becomes furrowed as it ages. Sharply climb out of Basswood Hollow to cross a paved road and drop into another hollow where a chimney stands. This is a relic of the Betsy Ross Cabin, which was built by Boy Scouts in the 1930s. Continue down the hollow past the cabin site to soon reach the beginning of the Mossy Ridge Loop. From here, backtrack a short distance to the Deep Well trailhead.

NEARBY/RELATED ACTIVITIES

The Warner Parks Nature Center is a point of pride for the Nashville park system. It offers wide-ranging environmental-education programs for visitors of all ages. Its large learning center has an exhibit hall, outdoor classroom, and more. Also in the area are a library with a large collection of natural-history books, a teaching pond, and a wildflower garden. For more information, visit **www .nashville.gov/parks/wpnc**.

10 PINNACLE TRAIL

KEY AT-A-GLANCE INFORMATION

LENGTH: 5 miles

CONFIGURATION: Loop

DIFFICULTY: Moderate

SCENERY: Hardwood and cedar forest

EXPOSURE: Mostly shady

TRAFFIC: Mountain bikers on weekends, quiet during the week

TRAIL SURFACE: Dirt, rocks, roots

HIKING TIME: 2.7 hours

ACCESS: No fees or permits

MAPS: Hamilton Creek Trails, available online at www.lrn.usace.army.mil/op/jpp/rec/hamilton.htm

FACILITIES: Restrooms, water at nearby Lakeside Trail parking area

IN BRIEF

This is a fun trail. If you are trying to get in one particular direction in a hurry, though, don't come here. This path twists, turns, winds, and comes back around on itself in an effort to make the most of the land in which it is located. The distance, along with numerous hills, will leave you feeling like you got your day's worth of exercise and enjoyed some solid Middle Tennessee scenery.

DESCRIPTION

If you are trying to follow where you are on the Pinnacle Trail by keeping up with the lay of the land, you may end up confused. This path doesn't necessarily go where you think it will or should go. That's because it is going nowhere, in particular, or everywhere, in general. Of all the trails I have ever hiked—and that is a lot—this is the most convoluted. On the plus side, the meandering trail extends the hike, so you might as well get your time's worth.

Leave the Pinnacle Trail parking area and cross the access road, passing a trail signboard. The trail courses along the edge of a field and enters the woods at the back of the field. Ascend a hill on a rooty trail, then drop back down on stairstep-like limestone outcrops. The trail then makes a hard left in a young

GPS Trailhead Coordinates

UTM Zone (WGS84) 16S

Easting 0533210

Northing 3995380

Latitude N 36° 6' 14.7"

Longitude W 86° 37' 51.7"

Directions

From Exit 219 on I-40 east of downtown Nashville, take Stewarts Ferry Pike south. Soon after leaving the interstate, Stewarts Ferry Road becomes Bell Road. Continue forward a total of 3.1 miles from the Interstate. Turn right on Ned Shelton Road and follow it 0.2 miles to a left turn into the Pinnacle trailhead parking area, on your left.

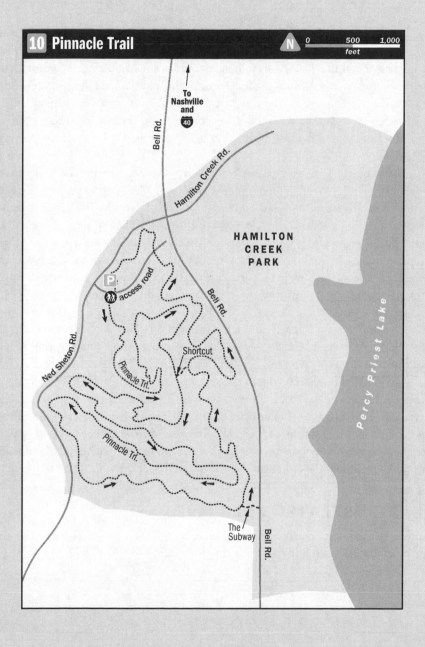

10 **Pinnacle Trail**

N   0   500   1,000
feet

To
Nashville
and
40

Bell Rd.

Hamilton Creek Rd.

HAMILTON
CREEK
PARK

Bell Rd.

access road

P

Ned Sheton Rd.

Pinnacle Trl.

Shortcut

Pinnacle Trl.

Pinnacle Trl.

Percy Priest Lake

The
Subway

Bell Rd.

forest and begins its seemingly ceaseless winding around as it heads up toward Beet Hill. You'll reach a trail junction at mile 1.2: the lesser-used trail leading left shortcuts the loop, and the Pinnacle Trail keeps right.

Pass occasional sinks in the hardwood forest. In one place the path splits, with the left fork dipping into a sink lined by rock bluffs and the right fork working around the bluffs. The paths join again, and soon you'll begin winding in and out of a brushy, open, and shaded forest. The path makes long and winding switchbacks covering all the land it can. At mile 2.5, enter an open field, staying on the left side of the field. You'll be in young woods before circling around the head of a hollow and nearing Ned Shelton Road, which will be off to your right at this point.

The Pinnacle Trail then passes beside a subdivision, nearing the backyards of houses. At mile 3.4, you'll come to a trail junction. The Subway goes to the right, heading beneath Bell Road and connecting to the Lakeside Trail (see page 32). The Pinnacle Trail goes to the left, passing through a planted pine grove. An old homesite lies beyond the pines. Look for bricks imbedded in the trail and other evidence of the old homes—and think of all the other homesites and artifacts that lie beneath the surface of nearby Percy Priest Lake. This part is formed on the shore of Priest Lake, and if it weren't for the lake, these homesites would be covered with houses.

At mile 3.8, you'll reach another trail junction. This is the other end of the loop shortcut. Immediately step over a small, narrow bridge and a spring branch. The trail undulates over small hills and swales, then enters a field broken with bushy cedar trees. Cross the closed access road. The trailhead is to the left on the access road, but don't take the shortcut if you want to hike the full 5 miles. Keep forward and pass some old piles of rock and rock walls from the days when these woods were a cleared farmstead. Circle back around toward the trailhead, walking by remnants of a brick-and-concrete block structure before reaching the trailhead at mile 5. That is the most convoluted walk you will ever do without getting lost.

NEARBY/RELATED ACTIVITIES

Hamilton Creek Park has picnic areas, lake access, BMX biking, mountain biking, and a sailboat marina. For more information, call (615) 862-8472.

SHELBY BOTTOMS NATURE PARK: EAST LOOP

11

IN BRIEF

The trails of Shelby Bottoms Nature Park were developed from west to east along the banks of the Cumberland River. The Nature Park offers paved greenways and primitive natural-surfaced trails. This less-traveled East Loop travels both surfaces as it winds among old fields, beneath the foliage of huge trees, in forestland, and by the river where Nashville was founded.

DESCRIPTION

This is a great hike for a crisp day during the cooler season. Much of the trail is in the open, which makes it prohibitively hot during summer. A weak winter sun, on the other hand, casting long shadows across fields and through barren trees, provides the best atmosphere at this nature park. The fields in this often-flooded bottomland were once tilled for crops,

KEY AT-A-GLANCE INFORMATION

LENGTH: 5.2 miles

CONFIGURATION: Loop

DIFFICULTY: Easy

SCENERY: Fields, woods, riverside

EXPOSURE: Mostly sunny

TRAFFIC: Quiet on weekdays, busy on weekends

TRAIL SURFACE: Asphalt, grass, dirt

HIKING TIME: 2.6 hours

ACCESS: No fees or permits

MAPS: Available at on Web at www .nashville.gov/greenways/images/ maps/shelbymetrocenter.jpg

FACILITIES: Water fountain at trailhead

Directions

From I-40 just east of downtown Nashville, take Exit 211B, then head west on I-24 to Exit 47A, Ellington Parkway/Spring Street (US 31A). Stay right beyond the Interstate, following Ellington Parkway. Exit Ellington Parkway onto Cleveland Street. Turn right on Cleveland Street, which becomes Eastland Avenue. Stay on Cleveland/Eastland 0.6 miles, then turn left on Gallatin Pike. Follow Gallatin Pike 1 mile to Cahal Avenue. Turn right on Cahal and follow it 1 mile, continuing forward as Cahal becomes Porter Avenue. Stay forward for 1 mile farther on Porter Avenue and intersect Rosebank Avenue. Turn left on Rosebank Avenue and soon turn right on Welcome Lane. Head just a short way on Welcome Lane, then turn left on Forest Green Drive to soon dead-end at the trailhead.

GPS Trailhead Coordinates

UTM Zone (WGS84) 16S

Easting 0526680

Northing 4005560

Latitude N 36° 11' 47.0"

Longitude W 86° 42' 11.2"

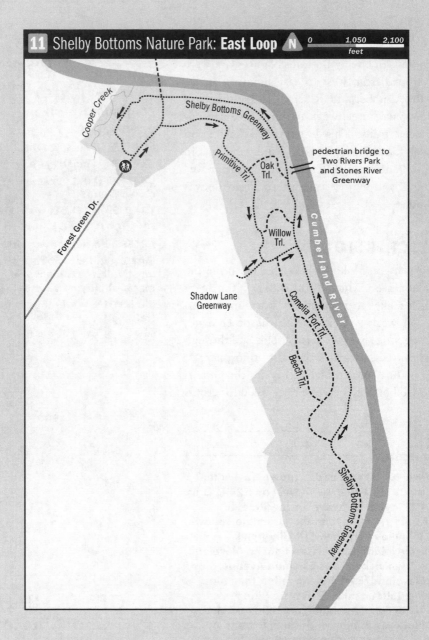

11 Shelby Bottoms Nature Park: **East Loop**

just as Native Americans did long before Nashville ever existed. Today, the park is being managed for wildlife. You will notice that many of the old fields are being allowed to revert into forest, and the transition is in many different stages. Patches of woodland are interspersed among the fields, most often along streambeds. Also scattered among the bottoms are large trees, which undoubtedly shaded the old farm buildings.

Leave the trailside kiosk after looking at the map. Various loop hikes are plentiful, but the following loop takes you through the most diverse terrain on the eastern side. Be apprised that most trail junctions are not marked, so pay close attention to avoid wandering around without knowing where you are.

Leave the Forest Green trailhead, and soon you'll intersect the Shelby Bottoms Greenway coming in from your left; this will be your return route. Stay forward, passing a sometimes-flooded wetland on your right. The terrain is mostly open as you keep along a wooded strip that was once a fence line. At 0.2 miles, turn right onto the gravel Primitive Trail, which soon loses its gravel and cruises along the old fence line. Ahead, you'll pass under two of the biggest hackberry trees in Middle Tennessee. Then curve right, where you'll see other old-growth trees in the area—chestnut, oak, and beech. Cut through a low wooded area, then climb to a field broken by occasional strips of woodland that shade intermittent streambeds. Cornelia Fort Airport is visible to your right.

As the Oak Trail turns left, keep forward in low brush, which, as evidenced by sycamore trees poking skyward, will eventually redevelop into forest. Watch for an unnamed trail, then the Willow Trail veering off to the left. Continue forward as the Primitive Trail turns right, then left, passing over a small, clear stream to meet the Shadow Lane Greenway at mile 1.3. This paved greenway heads left to meet the Shelby Bottoms Greenway and right to Shadow Lane. You, however, keep forward, crossing the paved greenway, and then veer left toward a bank of trees.

Now on the natural-surfaced Cornelia Fort Trail, you'll come alongside a tree bank and bisect a strip of woodland to reach a trail junction and sitting log. Turn right onto the Beech Trail and enter a rich hardwood forest of sweetgum, oak, and hackberry. Ahead, on the left, is a monstrous beech tree. Here, the Beech Trail intersects the Cornelia Fort Trail. Turn right and pass over a low, wet area rife with bamboo before emerging into open field and reaching the Shelby Bottoms Greenway at mile 2.4. Turn left on the paved path and begin the return leg of the loop.

You'll enter woodland and span a gullied streambed. The Cumberland River is to your right as the trail follows the wooded riverbank. Shortly bridge two more streambeds before again intersecting the Shadow Lane Greenway. The Shelby Bottoms Greenway keeps forward and descends to span another streambed on an iron trestle bridge. The trailside becomes more wooded, and the Willow Trail soon enters from the left. You stay on paved pathway, though. Dense stands of cane line the trail at times.

Soon you'll intersect the Oak Trail, but keep forward, staying on the greenway and passing the Cumberland River pedestrian bridge, which connects Shelby Bottoms to the Stones River Greenway. Wooded rock bluffs are visible on the far side of the Cumberland. The greenway bends north with the river as fields open to your left. At mile 4.7, a paved path, part of a short loop from the Forest Green trailhead, leaves left. In the future, another segment of the greenway will span the Cumberland River here. For now, though, keep forward, curving left along Cooper Creek and leaving the Cumberland. A watchful eye will notice a side trail leading right to a concrete-enclosed pipe that bridges Cooper Creek. The Shelby Bottoms Greenway shortly reaches the trail junction beside the trailhead. Turn right, walk a few steps, and complete the loop.

NEARBY/RELATED ACTIVITIES

Nearby Shelby Park offers a nature center, fishing, ball fields, tennis courts, and picnic grounds. The west side of Shelby Bottoms Nature Park also has trails.

SHELBY BOTTOMS NATURE PARK: WEST LOOP 12

IN BRIEF

Shelby Bottoms Nature Park, located on the banks of the Cumberland River just 3 miles from downtown Nashville, is the setting for this hike. Partly on paved greenway and partly on primitive trail, this loop traverses fields, woods, and riverside environments while circling the western edge of this park. Bird lovers will enjoy this walk, as the meadows, wooded edges, and bird boxes enhance avian life. Touch on Nashville history, as well, through the trailside interpretive information.

DESCRIPTION

At first glance, it is hard to believe such a large level area so close to downtown Nashville is undeveloped. But there is a reason—this riverside agglomeration of fields and woods is simply too close to the Cumberland River, which is always susceptible to flooding, and it thus has never been developed. The city of Nashville saw this 810-acre plot adjacent to Shelby Park as not only a valuable addition to the park system but also the absolute best use of the land. So, since 1997, Music City residents have been enjoying the paved and primitive

 KEY AT-A-GLANCE INFORMATION

LENGTH: 1.8 miles
CONFIGURATION: Loop
DIFFICULTY: Easy
SCENERY: Fields, woods, riparian environment
EXPOSURE: Mostly sunny
TRAFFIC: Steady, busy on weekends
TRAIL SURFACE: Asphalt, grass, mulch, gravel
HIKING TIME: 1 hour
ACCESS: No fees or permits
MAPS: Available at www.nashville.gov/greenways/images/maps/shelbymetrocenter.jpg
FACILITIES: Restrooms, water fountains at adjacent Shelby Park

Directions

From I-40 just east of downtown Nashville, take Exit 211B. Then head west on I-24 to Exit 49, Shelby Avenue/Coliseum. Head east on Shelby Avenue for just a short distance, then turn right on Fifth Street. Continue forward on Fifth Street 0.5 miles to Davidson Street. Turn left on Davidson Street and keep forward 1 mile to enter Shelby Park. Drive beyond the ball fields and keep right, making a right turn to pass under elevated railroad tracks. The parking area is just beyond the tracks.

GPS Trailhead Coordinates

UTM Zone (WGS84) 16S
Easting 0524740
Northing 4002220
Latitude N 36° 9' 57.3"
Longitude W 86° 43' 29.5"

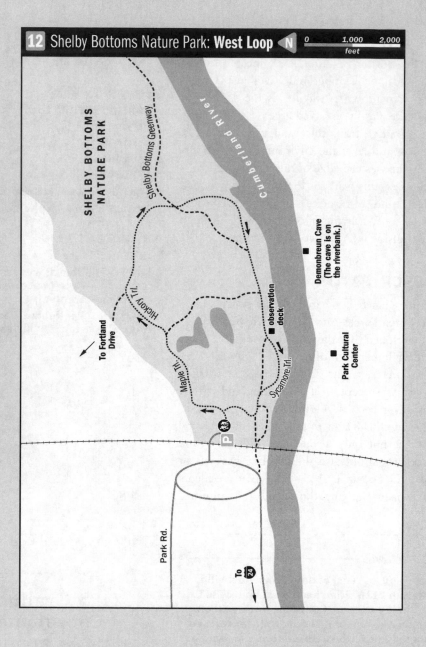

12 Shelby Bottoms Nature Park: **West Loop**

trails that wind through Shelby Bottoms.

Leave the parking area and pass a trailside kiosk. Ahead is a wooden bridge over a wetland. (Wetlands are scattered throughout the bottoms and are an important component of the park.) Ahead is a second kiosk with a good map of the bottoms. The trails are plotted on the kiosk map but not signed on the trails themselves.

Turn left on the paved Maple Trail, which is mostly devoid of trees because Shelby Bottoms has been cultivated by Nashvillians for generations. And why not? As the Cumberland River floods, it deposits rich sediment, making the bottoms a fertile place. Native Americans of a thousand years ago realized this and farmed the area's productive soil.

Pass through a strip of woodland. Beyond the strip, some fields are mowed, and others are growing up around you. Notice the young pine, maple, and sycamore trees. One day this path will be completely shaded. But for now, songbirds, deer, and other critters thrive in the edges between the woods and fields. There are also bird boxes scattered along the trail.

This path is currently so open overhead that it would not be fun to hike on a hot summer day. And the houses to your left are just above the floodplain and outside the park boundary.

Turn left again off the paved path onto the grassy Hickory Trail. This turn is just before an informative kiosk about Native Americans of the Nashville Basin. Pass a pedestrian access trail to Fortland Drive, where you'll come to a gravel trail; turn right here. Willow trees indicate a marsh on your left. The combination of marsh on one side of the trail and field on the other makes an excellent avian habitat. Don't be surprised if winged creatures burst forth from the high field grass and flap for the wooded marsh as you pass by.

Turn right onto the paved Shelby Bottoms Greenway, the master path of the nature park and the halfway point. Stay on it briefly, then turn left onto the Poplar Trail. Remember, the junctions are not marked but are easy to figure out. The trail is now shaded by a margin of woods along the riverbank. Watch for the side trail leading left to the river and a view of Demonbreun Cave across the Cumberland. This cave is named for the same man for whom the downtown Nashville street is named. Back in 1769, he actually spelled his name De Montbrun, but the spelling became corrupted along the way. Ol' De Montbrun hunted here and used the cave as a refuge from Native Americans. And his wife is said to have birthed the first child of European descent in Middle Tennessee in a nearby cave.

Keep forward on the paved path, and you'll reach a pierlike river overlook. The mini–castle structure you see in the middle of the river is part of the Nashville Waterworks complex across the river, which provides water for the city's residents. Built in 1892, the castlelike structure is a water-intake valve that's no longer functioning.

Leave the paved greenway just beyond the overlook for the Sycamore Trail. Overhead are tall sycamore, cottonwood, and hackberry trees. Enjoy the natural

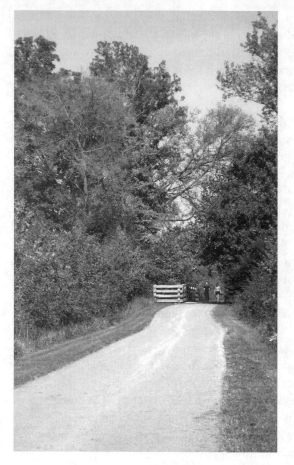

Shelby Bottoms Greenway winds through open and wooded areas.

environment down here, imagining the area as it was hundreds of years ago.

Soon you'll rejoin the paved greenway, where you'll find an informative board about exotic plants and birds that have helped create the landscape you see today. It makes you realize that the world has changed for good. Cross a bridge over a dry ravine, then turn right, passing by the trailhead kiosk to complete the loop.

NEARBY/RELATED ACTIVITIES

Nearby Shelby Park offers a nature center, fishing, ball fields, tennis courts, and picnic grounds. For more information, call (615) 862-8461.

SOUTH RADNOR LAKE LOOP 13

IN BRIEF

This hike winds through lush north-facing woods on the southern side of Radnor Lake State Park. The forest is rich with wildflowers in spring, is about as cool as the Middle Tennessee outdoors can get in summer, and offers a mosaic of color in fall. In winter, parts of this loop receive very little sun. Don't let the loop's short distance belie its challenging climbs, though.

DESCRIPTION

Get ready for a short but strenuous workout—but first you have to find the trailhead. The South Lake trailhead is not immediately evident from the nature center's parking area because it is a good way down Otter Creek Road. Leave the parking area and then walk around the car barriers on Otter Creek Road. Head uphill as the road bridges Otter Creek. You'll come to Radnor Lake Dam on your left. A side trail leads over the dam. Keep forward, and at 0.2 miles, on a left turn, reach the trailhead on the right side of Otter Creek Road.

Enter the woods, walk a few feet, and turn left on the South Lake Trail. Then begin walking easterly along the lower slope of a

KEY AT-A-GLANCE INFORMATION

LENGTH: 2.5 miles
CONFIGURATION: Loop
DIFFICULTY: Moderate
SCENERY: Lush hardwood forest
EXPOSURE: Very shady
TRAFFIC: Fairly busy, especially on weekends
TRAIL SURFACE: Dirt, rocks
HIKING TIME: 1.5 hours
ACCESS: No fees or permits required
MAPS: Available on the Web at www.state.tn.us/environment/parks/RadnorLake
FACILITIES: Restrooms, water at nature center

Directions

From Exit 78 on I-65 south of downtown Nashville, take Harding Place Road west 2.2 miles to Granny White Pike; along the way, Harding Place Road becomes Battery Lane. Turn left on Granny White Pike and follow it 1.7 miles to Otter Creek Road. Turn left on Otter Creek Road and drive 0.3 miles to the parking area on the left. The South Lake Trail starts 0.2 miles down the closed portion of Otter Creek Road beyond the parking area.

GPS Trailhead Coordinates

UTM Zone (WGS84) 16S
Easting   0524740
Northing 4002220
Latitude   N 36° 9' 57.3"
Longitude   W 86° 43' 29.5"

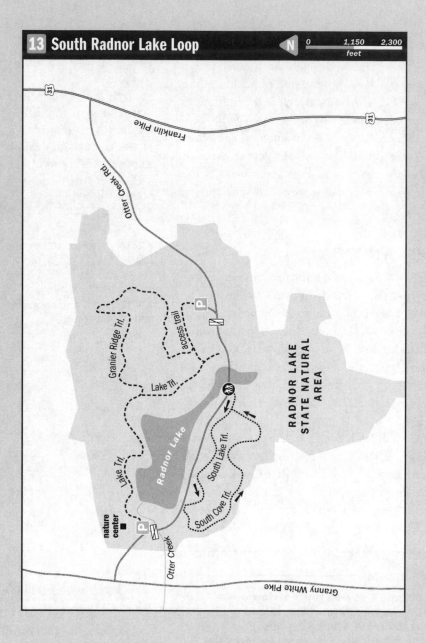

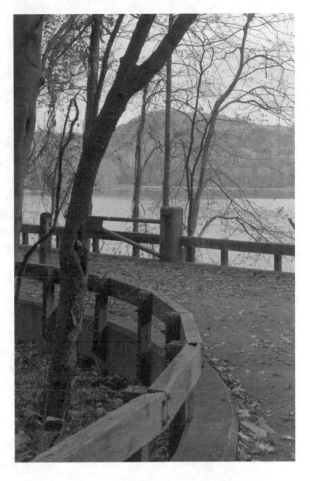

Wooded hills rise across scenic Radnor Lake.

surprisingly steep hill. These are known as the Overton Hills, even though they lie within the town-limit boundaries of Forest Hills, an enclave now enveloped by the city of Nashville. Travel beneath a hardwood forest of maple and oak, and Radnor Lake, 85 acres in size, is off to your left. This lake was impounded in 1914 by the Louisville and Nashville (L&N) Railroad to furnish water for their steam engines and livestock at the nearby long-disappeared Radnor Yards. This lake initially was a private hunting and fishing preserve for L&N officials. Shortly after the lake was impounded, both native and migratory birds began using the lake.

L&N officials realized the natural importance of the lake and declared the lake a wildlife sanctuary at the request of the Tennessee Ornithological Society.

Ascend the steep hillside. It's so steep, in fact, that wooden berms have been placed on the downside of the trail to keep it level and prevent erosion. Numerous downed trees lie in various states of decay, and it's easy to see the slow but sure cycle of plant life here. It may take a hundred years or more for a tree to grow robust and tall, before wind, lightning, or disease strikes it down. Then the tree lies upon the ground for decades, slowly rotting and serving as a home and a food source for nature's smaller critters and bugs. But the very richness of the decay will someday feed another tree growing in its place. And so the cycle goes, extending through many human lifetimes.

Work back down toward Radnor Lake along a dry drainage area, passing some sizable oaks. Also, notice the deeply fissured trunks of locust trees. These pioneer trees grow in disturbed or cleared areas. The short-lived locust grows rapidly and provides shade for less-sun-tolerant trees, such as sugar maple, then falls and provides nutrients for the trees that follow.

Ahead, a small pond filled with bright-green duck moss lies between the hillside and Otter Creek Road. Circle around the pond, as a side trail leads down to Otter Creek Road. Soon you'll reach a trail junction at mile 1. The South Lake Trail keeps forward, but you turn right and take the South Cove Trail. Immediately, head up a tough hill then swing around a cove. In this area the woods are tangled with vines.

Bridge a ravine and begin switchbacking up a hill, meeting an old woods road at some wide steps. Soon, top out on the ridgeline, with its obscured views to the north and south at mile 1.6. The trail splits here. To the left, the old road heads a short distance to one of the many contemplation benches set along the path. The main trail swings around a rib ridge with shagbark hickories and thick ground cover. Return shortly to the main ridgeline. Then descend on the old woods road into a tangle of thick woods in the heart of a cove, which sees very little sun. You'll soon meet the South Lake Trail. Walk a few feet to Otter Creek Road and backtrack to the nature center.

NEARBY/RELATED ACTIVITIES

Be sure to stop in the visitor center before or after this hike. It offers an excellent slide show available upon request as well as other nature displays. For more information, call (615) 373-3467 or visit **www.tnstateparks.com.**

STONES RIVER GREENWAY OF NASHVILLE

14

IN BRIEF

Murfreesboro developed the first greenway along the Stones River, but Nashville is giving them a run for their money with this scenic gem that begins just below Percy Priest Dam and runs along the Stones in a real mix of attractive settings. The trail has now been extended to Two Rivers Park near the Cumberland River.

DESCRIPTION

Like most of you readers who've visited this area, I have driven I-40 past Percy Priest Dam and have seen the large flat and spillway next to the Interstate. It's easy to tell by the many cars parked there that fishing is popular. But upon taking the Stones River Greenway, which follows the once-again-free-flowing Stones River, I realized it's also a great place to take a walk.

The track, about 8 feet wide and paved, heads away from the dam. Before leaving the area, though, you may want to check out the fishermen trying their best to get a lunker out of the dam spillway, where the Stones River is once again free to flow to meet the Cumberland River. Pass underneath the double bridges of I-40, and you'll soon leave the noise behind. Because the Stones River flows from the bottom

KEY AT-A-GLANCE INFORMATION

LENGTH: 6 miles
CONFIGURATION: There-and-back
DIFFICULTY: Moderate
SCENERY: Woods, fields, riverside
EXPOSURE: Part sun, part shade
TRAFFIC: Moderate to heavy on weekends
TRAIL SURFACE: Paved
HIKING TIME: 2.5 hours
ACCESS: No fees or permits
MAPS: Available on the Web at www.nashville.gov/greenways/ images/maps/stonesriver.jpg
FACILITIES: Restrooms and picnic area at nearby Percy Priest Dam Army Corps of Engineers visitor center
SPECIAL COMMENTS: Percy Priest Dam has fishing, picnicking, and all the pleasures of a big lake behind it. Visit the Army Corps of Engineers Web site at www.lrn .usace.army.mil/op/jpp/rec for more information.

Directions

From Exit 219 on I-40, east of downtown Nashville, take Stewarts Ferry Pike south 0.2 miles to Bell Road. Turn left on Bell Road and follow it to an intersection. The right turn is into the Percy Priest Dam visitor center. Take the left turn at this intersection, dropping down to a large, level area below the dam. The Stones River Greenway begins at the northern end of the parking area, toward I-40.

GPS Trailhead Coordinates

UTM Zone (WGS84) 16S
Easting   0534140
Northing   4001340
Latitude   N 36° 9' 28.4"
Longitude   W 86° 37' 14.0"

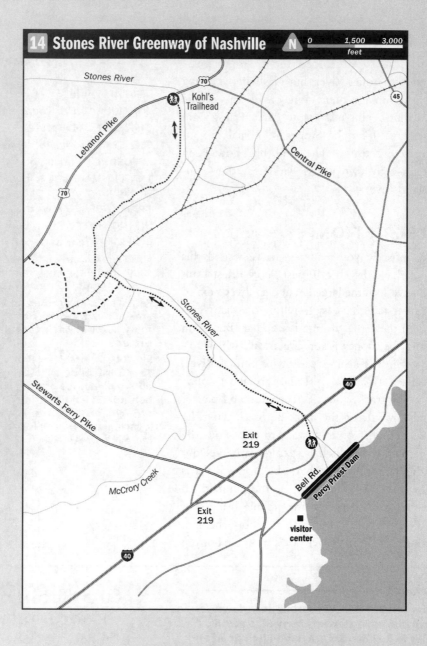

14 Stones River Greenway of Nashville   N   0   1,500   3,000
feet

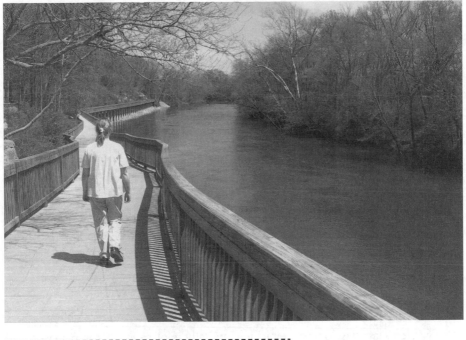

A hiker travels a bridge bordering the bluffs of the Stones River.

of the lake through the dam, it is normally clear, green—and cold! Notice attractive bluffs across the river and a wooden fence that stands between the river and the greenway.

Even when the greenway doesn't border the river, short gravel-and-dirt tracks lead to the water's edge. At 0.5 miles, a paved path leads left and uphill to an adjoining neighborhood. And at 0.7 miles, the path reaches a particularly scenic area. Here, the path bridges McCrory Creek, a beautiful blue stream that still exemplifies the coloration of many creeks in Middle Tennessee. Here, the slow waters wind to meet the Stones River. A path leads right to a hilly overlook of McCrory Creek and onward to the actual confluence of McCrory Creek and the Stones River. Take the time to explore this little locale.

Continue beyond the bridge, and the trail opens to a field. Here, a parallel track runs through the grassland, and the greenway turns to dip into fully shaded thick woods along the Stones River. Notice the large sycamores along the river. At 1 mile, the trail passes two concrete structures that I believe were water-gauging stations. The trail then reenters a field and continues downstream to span a smaller branch on a steel truss bridge at 1.4 miles. The creek here cuts a steep, deep valley for its size. Just ahead, you can see the cut-stone abutments of an old bridge spanning the Stones River. A dirt track leading right heads to the base of one abutment and allows you to see another abutment standing silently in the river. You'll notice a cedar tree growing from the top of this pillar.

The greenway passes under a railroad bridge before making its big climb, and the path turns uphill to reach the top of a bluff over the river. Top out at 1.8 miles and pass under some power lines before descending to the river and the highlight of the greenway. After skirting on the edge of some condos, the greenway works its way downstream along a bridge that runs parallel to the river bluffs. From this bridge, walkers can gain great views up and down the Stones.

The bridge rejoins terra firma at 2.2 miles, and the greenway keeps near the Stones, crossing intermittent streambeds west of the river. Near Lebanon Pike, the trail turns uphill to reach what is commonly called the Kohl's trailhead, ending at 2.9 miles. This trailhead is in a shopping-center parking lot near the Kohl's store off Lebanon Pike, east of Briley Parkway. Most greenway users simply backtrack to the dam trailhead. The greenway continues onward to border the Cumberland River near its confluence with the Stones at Heartland Park, where there is a trailhead. Another trailhead is located at Two Rivers Park. A pedestrian bridge across the Cumberland River has been constructed, connecting Shelby Bottoms Greenway to the Stones River Greenway.

NEARBY/RELATED ACTIVITIES

Percy Priest Dam has fishing, picnicking, and all the pleasures of a big lake behind it. The Stones River makes for a fine 7-mile trip to the Cumberland River with a takeout at Peeler Park boat ramp. Visit the Army Corps of Engineers Web site at **www.lrn.usace.army.mil/op/jpp/rec** for more information.

VOLUNTEER-DAY LOOP 15

IN BRIEF

This hike explores the wilder side of Long Hunter State Park. Follow Volunteer Trail a half mile through the woods and pick up the Day Loop Trail, which skirts the rocky shoreline of Percy Priest Lake. Circle around to a high bluff and enjoy stunning lake views before reaching a quiet cove that was once settled. Ramble over a hill filled with tall oaks, then backtrack a half mile to finish the hike.

DESCRIPTION

The state of Tennessee is very fortunate to be in control of this parkland that covers some 33 shoreline miles of Percy Priest Lake. As Nashville has expanded and lakeshore property has become more desirable for housing, the value of this land has skyrocketed. In fact, to obtain this shoreline now would break the state's budget. The property is currently under a 99-year lease from the U.S. Army Corps of Engineers, which dammed Percy Priest Lake in 1968. Long Hunter State Park was established shortly after the damming.

And how pretty this trail is, running along the shore, over limestone outcrops, through stream sheds, and around peninsulas jutting into the lake. Start your hike on the white-blazed Volunteer Trail, named for Boy Scout

KEY AT-A-GLANCE INFORMATION

LENGTH: 4 miles
CONFIGURATION: Loop
DIFFICULTY: Moderate
SCENERY: Hardwood and cedar forest, rock bluffs, lake views
EXPOSURE: Nearly all shady
TRAFFIC: Busy on weekends
TRAIL SURFACE: Dirt, rocks, leaves
HIKING TIME: 2.1 hours
ACCESS: No fees or permits required
MAPS: Available on the Web at www.state.tn.us/environment/parks/gis/pdf/printmaps/longhunter.pdf
FACILITIES: None
SPECIAL COMMENTS: Volunteer Trail continues to a backcountry campsite. The Bakers Grove Recreation Area part of Long Hunter State Park is primitive, but the Couchville Unit of the state park has a visitor center, picnic area, rental canoes, and more trails. For more information, call (615) 885-2422 or visit www.tnstateparks.com.

Directions

From Exit 226 on I-40 east of downtown Nashville, take South Mount Juliet Road, TN 171, south 4.2 miles. Veer right at the split as TN 171 becomes Hobson Pike. Keep forward 1.8 miles farther, turning right on Bakers Grove Lane. Drive just a short distance, then turn left on Bakers Grove Road and follow it a short distance to the parking area at the dead end.

GPS Trailhead Coordinates

UTM Zone (WGS84) 16S
Easting 0540270
Northing 3995270
Latitude N 36° 6' 11.1"
Longitude W 86° 33' 9.1"

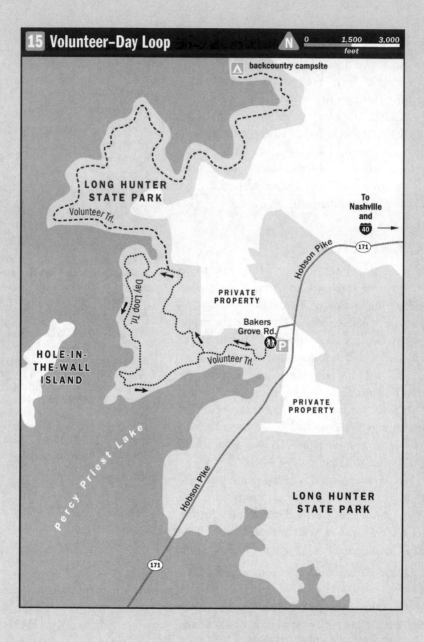

15 Volunteer–Day Loop

N

0   1,500   3,000
feet

backcountry campsite

LONG HUNTER
STATE PARK

Volunteer Trl.

To
Nashville
and
40 →

Hobson Pike

171

Day Loop Trl.

PRIVATE
PROPERTY

Bakers
Grove Rd.

P

HOLE-IN-
THE-WALL
ISLAND

Volunteer Trl.

PRIVATE
PROPERTY

Percy Priest Lake

LONG HUNTER
STATE PARK

Hobson Pike

171

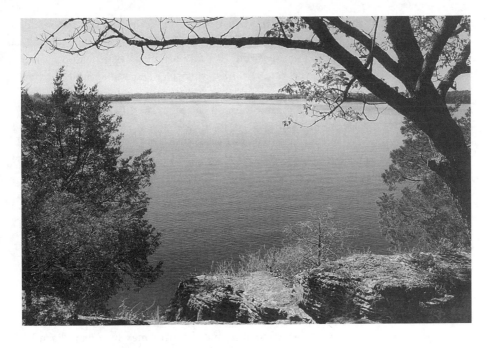

Bluff-top view of Percy Priest Lake

volunteers who constructed the path. Walk down an old gravel road flanked with brush. Off to your right is an overgrown fence line, and the sky is open overhead. Soon you'll leave the roadbed and turn right into a forest carpeted with vinca minor, also known as cemetery ivy. Not surprisingly, this was once a burial place. The Corps of Engineers relocated the cemetery when the dam was built. You'll pass a small sinkhole to the right of the trail. Keep forward to reach a footbridge with handrails; it spans a wet-weather drainage area that forms the lake cove visible to your left.

The path picks and twists its way amid a rock jumble before reaching a junction at 0.6 miles. Turn left on the orange-blazed Day Loop Trail, immediately stepping over a dry wash. Stay along the shoreline in a young forest. The trail here runs alongside a limestone rampart running parallel to the shoreline, zigzagging through the rocks, sometimes above the rampart, sometimes below. At mile 1, the path nears Percy Priest Lake. Walk a few feet to the shoreline.

You are now looking over the Stones River Valley, which was flooded to create Percy Priest Lake. The Stones River was named for Uriah Stone, a long hunter of yesteryear. When explorers, settlers, and hunters began pouring westward over the Appalachian Mountains in the mid-1700s, some of them would explore the fringes of settled land and Native American territory for extended periods that became known as "long hunts." During periods lasting up to a year, the hunters would acquire hides and furs of deer, beaver, elk, and otters, then return east to sell them. These men, who made their living in the fur trade, became known as long hunters.

Uriah Stone favored the hunting grounds of a particular river heading south from the Cumberland River. On one trip near this river, he was double-crossed by a Frenchman with whom he had partnered, who stole his hides. Other long hunters named the Stones River after him as a result of this episode. Consequently, 200 years later, Long Hunter State Park was named for the Stones River valley that it abuts.

Turn away from the lake at mile 1.1 and notice small sinks and rock outcrops amid the thick woodland area. The trail makes a sharp U-turn near an old fence line, then returns to the lake's edge. Here, you can look west across the lake at a rock bluff on Hole-in-the-Wall Island. To your right, in the distance, is the shoreline along which the Volunteer Trail continues to a backcountry campsite. Cruise along the shoreline and soon you'll reach a small pond separated from the lake by only a thin strip of trees.

The shoreline steepens and the trail climbs, reaching a bluffline that offers dramatic views. Watch your step here among the rocks. Eventually, leave the bluffline and head farther inland. Turn away from the lake, ascending alongside a deep, dry creekbed. Piles of rocks indicate that this area may have been farmed at one time. Turn back downstream on the dry creekbed and intersect the Volunteer Trail at a second dry drainage at mile 2.7. Just across the drainage, to the left, are an information board and the trek to the backcountry campsite. Turn right on the Volunteer Trail, begin climbing along this drainage, and pass an old stone fence at mile 2.8. Keep ascending over a wooded hill. Make a hard right at mile 3.1, briefly picking up an old woods road. Soon, turn left off of the old road to make a prolonged descent along a streambed. Cross this streambed to reach a familiar junction at mile 3.4. Stay forward, as the Day Loop Trail you already hiked leaves right, and retrace your steps 0.6 miles to the trailhead.

WARNER WOODS TRAIL 16

IN BRIEF

Big trees, deep woods, and a good view are all rolled into one hike located less than 10 air miles from downtown Nashville. This loop hike traverses land set aside by Luke Lea for a park near the town of Belle Meade, now enveloped by greater Nashville. Hikers will pass several large, old-growth trees amid a rich forest and Luke Lea Heights, which offers a far-reaching view of the Nashville Basin, downtown Nashville, and beyond.

DESCRIPTION

While on your hike, you might want to thank Percy Warner, who was chairman of the Nashville Park Board in the 1920s. Warner's son-in-law, Luke Lea, was in the process of developing what would later become the town of Belle Meade when Warner convinced Lea to donate some of his land for this park. Percy Warner died suddenly after this deal was made, and the park was named for him. Adjacent Edwin Warner Park is named for Warner's brother who became the next park-board chairman. The current total acreage of these two parks is 2,684 acres, 2,058 of which are in Percy Warner Park.

Begin the Warner Woods Trail behind the covered trail-map kiosk, and trace the

KEY AT-A-GLANCE INFORMATION

LENGTH: 2.5 miles
CONFIGURATION: Loop
DIFFICULTY: Easy to moderate
SCENERY: Rich hillside woods and views
EXPOSURE: Shady
TRAFFIC: Moderate, somewhat busy on weekends
TRAIL SURFACE: Dirt, roots
HIKING TIME: A little more than an hour
ACCESS: No fees or permits
MAPS: Available on the Web at www.nashville.gov/parks/images/previous/percywarner_map.gif
FACILITIES: Portable bathroom at trailhead
SPECIAL COMMENTS: Stay with the white blazes, as there are many trail junctions.

Directions

From the point where TN 100 begins at US 70 near the Belle Meade post office, head west on TN 100 1.7 miles to the large stone gates on the left that mark the Deep Well entrance of Percy Warner Park. Turn left off TN 100 and pass through the gates, staying right when the road splits. Reach the Deep Well trailhead parking at 0.6 miles. The Warner Woods Trail starts behind the trailside kiosk.

GPS Trailhead Coordinates

UTM Zone (WGS84)   16S
Easting   0533720
Northing   3995490
Latitude   N 36° 6' 17.9"
Longitude   W 86° 37' 31.2"

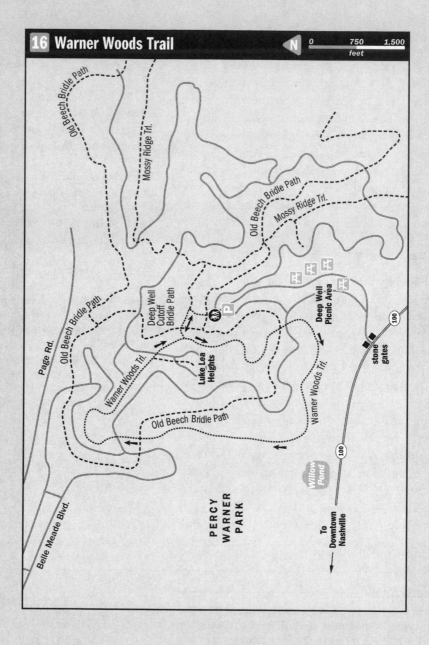

16 Warner Woods Trail

N   0   750   1,500
                            feet

Old Beech Bridle Path

Mossy Ridge Trl.

Old Beech Bridle Path

Mossy Ridge Trl.

Old Beech Bridle Path

Page Rd.

Deep Well Cutoff Bridle Path

Deep Well Picnic Area

Warner Woods Trl.

Luke Lea Heights

Old Beech Bridle Path

Warner Woods Trl.

stone gates

100

100

Belle Meade Blvd.

PERCY WARNER PARK

Willow Pond

To Downtown Nashville

white-blazed path forward to immediately cross the Old Beech Bridle Path. Keep forward, climbing a hill, and reach another junction. Here the red-blazed Mossy Ridge Trail goes off to the right, and the white-blazed Warner Woods Trail goes to the left. Turn left, looking up on the hillside to your right beyond the junction for a giant white oak. Soon cross the Deep Well Cutoff Bridle Path, continue forward, passing a huge tulip tree, and reach the loop portion of the Warner Woods Trail. Turn left and begin to swing around a knob of the Harpeth Hills, climbing through rich, vine-draped woods to reach Farrell Road.

Actually a remnant of the scenic driving roads that course through this park, Farrell Road was never paved, as the remaining scenic roads are today, and has reverted to a rough dirt path. Maples and tulip trees are reclaiming the margins of the way, further diminishing its appearance as a road. Another notable tree in the area is the shagbark hickory, which has an easily identifiable bark that appears to be peeling.

At 0.8 miles, you'll cross a paved scenic road and enter Buggy Hollow. An intermittent stream sometimes flows here to feed Willow Pond, the body of water beside TN 100. Pass a contemplation bench looking over the remains of a big white oak that is but a skeleton of its former self. Its limbs are slowly falling off, but it will be beyond our lifetimes before this giant has completely returned to the earth. Come alongside a second contemplation bench in Buggy Hollow adjacent to the intermittent streambed; many exotic vines cling to the trunks of the trees here. Cross the bridle path again and a paved road at mile 1.7. Not far from here, a side trail leads left down to the palatial main entrance to Percy Warner Park at the end of Belle Meade Boulevard.

The trail then climbs a bit to Hairpin Curve, so named for a turn in the scenic road the trail nears. The crumbled stone wall along the road is evidence that at least one auto didn't make the curve. The Warner Woods Trail curves a lot less than the road and keeps ascending toward Luke Lea Heights, reaching a paved road at mile 2.1. Turn right and walk about 50 yards, where the road splits. Look for the foot trail between the two roads that leads straight up the ridgeline. Take this path to shortly emerge at Luke Lea Summit, where a view to the northeast opens up beside a couple of cedar benches. Look to the horizon at downtown Nashville and beyond across the Nashville Basin. This 920-foot knob offers an impressive view of Downtown Nashville, which lies around 400 feet in elevation. Backtrack to where the Warner Woods Trail crossed the scenic drive and head downhill, reaching the end of the trail's loop portion at 2.4 miles. From this point, backtrack 0.1 miles to the Deep Well trailhead.

NEARBY/RELATED ACTIVITIES

The Deep Well Picnic Area has many fine picnic shelters, so consider combining a cookout or outdoor lunch with your hike. For more information, call (615) 352-6299 or visit **www.nashville.gov/parks/wpnc**.

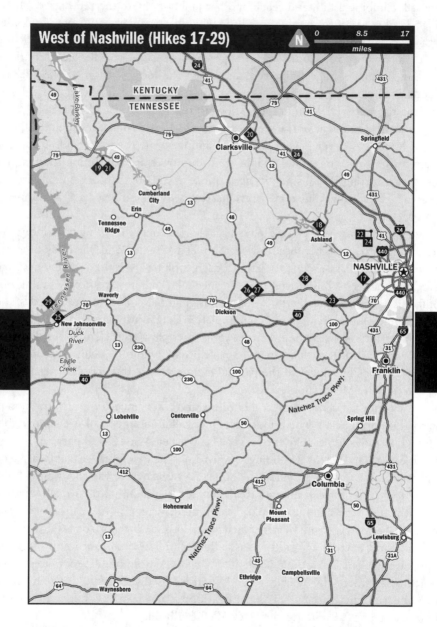

West of Nashville (Hikes 17-29)

KENTUCKY
TENNESSEE

Lake Barkley

Clarksville

Springfield

Cumberland City

Erin

Tennessee Ridge

Ashland

NASHVILLE

Waverly

Dickson

New Johnsonville

Duck River

Eagle Creek

Lobelville

Centerville

Franklin

Natchez Trace Pkwy;

Spring Hill

Columbia

Hohenwald

Mount Pleasant

Lewisburg

Natchez Trace Pkwy;

Ethridge

Campbellsville

Waynesboro

17 Bells Bend Loop 74

18 Cumberland River Bicentennial Trail...... 78

19 Confederate Earthworks Walk 81

20 Dunbar Cave State Natural Area Loop 85

21 Fort Donelson Battlefield Loop............ 88

22 Henry Hollow Loop 92

23 Hidden Lake Double Loop 96

24 Highland Trail at Beaman Park........... 100

25 Johnsonville State Historic Area Loop 104

26 Montgomery Bell Northeast Loop 108

27 Montgomery Bell Southwest Loop........ 111

28 Narrows of Harpeth Hike 116

29 Nathan Bedford Forrest Five Mile Loop... 120

WEST
INCLUDING ASHLAND CITY, CLARKSVILLE, AND DICKSON

17 BELLS BEND LOOP

KEY AT-A-GLANCE INFORMATION

LENGTH: 2.6 miles
CONFIGURATION: Loop
DIFFICULTY: Easy
SCENERY: Open fields, Cumberland River floodplain, bluffs
EXPOSURE: Mostly sunny
TRAFFIC: Moderate on weekends
TRAIL SURFACE: Gravel, grass, a little asphalt
HIKING TIME: 1.3 hours
ACCESS: No fees or permits
MAPS: Available at www.nashville .gov/greenways
FACILITIES: Nature Center near trailhead, variable hours

IN BRIEF

Bells Bend Park is the setting for this loop hike along the banks of the Cumberland River. It travels through rolling fields and alongside the big river, where you can enjoy vistas of hills and bluffs before returning to the trailhead. Opened in 2007, the park also has a nature center.

DESCRIPTION

Talk about turning bad into good. The city of Nashville purchased the Bells Bend area back in 1989 for use as a landfill. Luckily, former mayor Bill Purcell had other ideas for this scenic tract on the banks of the Cumberland, and two decades later we have a scenic park with hiking trails. Now the 800-plus-acre tract of land is a mix of woods and open areas set along a picturesque arc of land west of downtown. The former farmland still has wooded fence lines, old farm ponds, and even a barn. Nonetheless, the park is a green oasis, and its natural amenities are being enhanced. Keep in mind that shade is limited, so this may not be a desirable summertime trek.

Leave the parking area and trailhead and immediately cross an intermittent creek on an iron bridge. The gravel track cuts across a field and then two lines of trees to reach a trail

GPS Trailhead Coordinates

UTM Zone (WGS 84) 16S
Easting   0506638
Northing   4001054
Latitude   N 36° 9' 22.0"
Longitude W 86° 55' 34.2"

Directions ⟶

From Exit 24 on Briley Parkway northwest of downtown, take TN 12 west 3 miles to Old Hickory Boulevard. Turn left onto Old Hickory Boulevard and follow it 4.2 miles to the right turn into Bells Bend Park. Follow this road to dead-end at the trailhead in 0.1 mile.

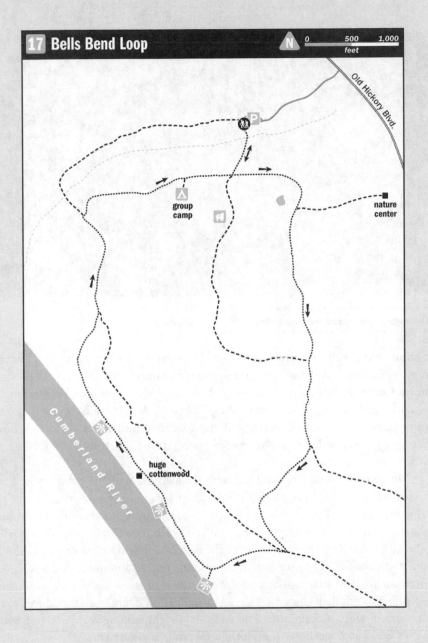

17 Bells Bend Loop

N

0   500   1,000
feet

Old Hickory Blvd.

group camp

nature center

Cumberland River

huge cottonwood

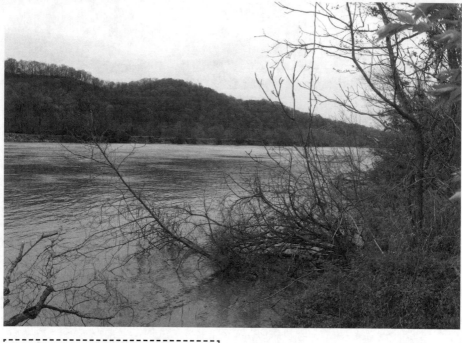

The mighty Cumberland arcs past Bells Bend.

junction at 0.1 mile. Here, extremely wide grassy tracks branch to the left and right, while the gravel trail continues straight. Head left (easterly). Bells Bend Nature Center stands atop a hill in the distance. This is easily the widest trail in this entire guidebook, perhaps extending 12 feet wide. You don't quite make the nature center, as the trail curves south and reaches a junction at 0.3 miles. Continue straight as another super-wide trail leads left to the nature center. Note the trailside pond.

The loop continues meandering south through fields of grass and briers. Lines of trees delineate the fields, while the hills and bluffs of the Cumberland River rise in the distance. The open landscape lies bare the contours of the land. At 0.6 miles, a shortcut trail leads right, toward the trailhead. Here you'll reach the highest point of the hike, with views stretching out to the back and beyond. One thing you'll note is the prevalence of cell towers, radio towers, and other communication towers that reflect our modern life. Pass through another line of trees at 0.7 miles and begin descending to another junction. Here, a combination of trails and old farm roads make a mini-loop of their own. This hike stays right, aiming for the Cumberland River. Cedars and hackberry trees form a tree line to your right.

At 1.1 miles, intersect the aforementioned mini-loop. Keep shooting for the big water, as yet another trail runs the margin between the floodplain and the hills. You are now in the river floodplain, which comprises 30 percent of this park. Soon you'll come to the river, where a screen of cane and trees grows along the banks. A spur trail leads down to a view of the river, and a mud trail descends to the water's edge. The mud trail was created by dogs—and a few humans—who just can't fight the lure of the water. Travel northwest along the mighty Cumberland, which flows strongly to meet the Ohio River. At 1.4 miles, pass another river clearing. The bluffs across the river rise nearly 400 feet from the water. Most of the trees along the river's edge are small, but you do pass a huge cottonwood at 1.5 miles. It looks old enough to have seen a Native American float by in a dugout canoe.

Climb away from the river and pass the other end of the trail that runs along the floodplain at 1.9 miles. Continue heading toward the trailhead, passing a trail that leads left to cross the stream passing near the trailhead. The main trail heads east and meets the park's group camp at 2.4 miles. Keep straight here to reach another junction and the loop's end at 2.5 miles. Turn left here, backtracking to the trailhead, and complete your hike at 2.6 miles. Just think, this could've been a landfill.

NEARBY/RELATED ACTIVITIES

Bells Bend Nature Center is located at the park. It is currently open Tuesday and Thursday from noon until 4 p.m. and Saturday from 9 a.m. until 4 p.m. For more information, visit **www.nashville.gov/parks/nature.**

18 CUMBERLAND RIVER BICENTENNIAL TRAIL

KEY AT-A-GLANCE INFORMATION

LENGTH: 8 miles

CONFIGURATION: There-and-back

DIFFICULTY: Moderate

SCENERY: Hardwood forest, creek embayment, small creeks

EXPOSURE: Mostly shady

TRAFFIC: Some on weekends, but not too busy

TRAIL SURFACE: Pea gravel, grass, rocks, asphalt

HIKING TIME: 3.5 hours

ACCESS: No fees or permits

MAPS: Available by calling (615) 792-4211

FACILITIES: Restrooms, picnic tables at trailhead and along the way

SPECIAL COMMENTS: The rail-trail extends beyond this segment.

IN BRIEF

This rustic rail-trail quietly runs through a rural section of the lower Cumberland River. The path is flanked by bluffs on one side and water on the other. Look for wildlife.

DESCRIPTION

Ashland City did the right thing by converting the old tracks of the Tennessee Central Railroad into a path that is now enjoyed by nature lovers of all stripes. The valley of the Cumberland River is wide at the point along which the rail-trail travels. To prevent its tracks from flooding, the railroad had built a right-of-way along the northern edge of the river valley. Steep bluffs to the north and a vast floodplain to the south border the trail. The Cumberland River is just out of sight, but the embayment of Sycamore Creek, which flows into the Cumberland, lies along much of the rail-trail, lending a watery aspect. Cheatham Dam, downstream on the Cumberland, creates the embayment.

The railroad-turned-greenway passes over small creeks that have cut their way through the riverside bluffs. Here, trestles bridge the creeks, offering a bird's-eye view of the surroundings. In places the right-of-way has been elevated to keep the former tracks level. The

GPS Trailhead Coordinates

UTM Zone (WGS84) 16S

Easting   0492950

Northing   4015360

Latitude   N 36° 17' 6.5"

Longitude   W 87° 4' 42.4"

Directions

From Exit 188 on Interstate 40 west of downtown Nashville, take TN 249 north and stay with it 17 miles to reach TN 49. Turn right onto TN 49 east, and cross the Cumberland River to reach Ashland City and TN 12 in 1 mile. Turn left on TN 12, and follow it north 1.1 miles to Chapmansboro Road. Turn left on Chapmansboro Road, and follow it 0.1 mile to the Marks Creek trailhead on your right.

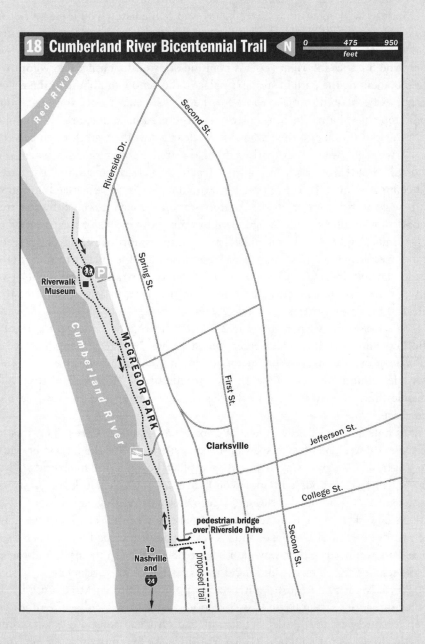

path's flatness makes it appealing for those who want to concentrate on seeing the sights around them, rather than huffing and puffing through hills.

Start by walking around a metal gate, and immediately you'll pass a trailside kiosk and picnic table. A hardwood forest of sycamore, oak, and sweetgum trees shades the path. Look for railroad ties and occasional steel rails near the greenway, where you'll notice informative signs pointing out specific bushes and wildflowers that bloom along the path in spring. In places, the yellow-tan bluffs to the right of the trail were blasted to make room for the tracks; cedar trees hang precariously from atop these bluffs. In other places, small creeks have cut through the bluffs and formed little valleys; their waters flow clear below the trail through culverts.

A wooded swamp lies to the left of the trail; farther on, this watery area becomes a full-fledged lake. At mile 1.1, reach the Turkey Junction native gardens and comfort station. To the left are a restroom and a garden encircled by a gravel path. Wastewater flows from the comfort station through a wetland-water-treat-ment-demonstration system. A signboard explains how the water treatment works.

Cumberland River Bicentennial Trail continues northwest, passing a second trestle over a small creek at mile 1.4. Here, a side trail leads left to picnic tables beside the Sycamore Creek embayment. The trail straddles the right-of-way between the lake on the left and the bluff on the right, passing a third trestle at mile 1.8. Pass a longer trestle at mile 2.2.

The tree canopy opens by mile 2.4 as an old roadbed goes to the right up a hollow. Soon you'll reach a bridge that stretches 200 feet in length above the embayment, and farm country—old wooden outbuildings, fields, rows of trees—is visible around you. Hills rise on the far side of the Cumberland River. The trailside bluff gives way beyond this last bridge, giving the greenway a more open feel.

At mile 3.2, you'll reach the trestle spanning Sycamore Creek. This trestle is curved and has a steel-frame span in its center; it is by far the largest bridge on the rail-trail. The greenway is paved in asphalt beyond this final bridge. Keep forward in thick woods and soon you'll reach a trailside kiosk and restroom. Turn right and drop off the elevated right-of-way to reach Chapmansboro Road and the end of this greenway segment. The east side of the road identifies this as the Sycamore Harbor trailhead, and the west side of the road identifies it as the Eagle Pass trailhead. Either way, you have reached the 4-mile mark and the end of this segment. Cheatham Dam is 2.5 miles farther on the greenway.

If you want to hike just 4 miles to this point and not backtrack, use the fol-lowing directions to the Eagle Pass–Sycamore Harbor trailhead at the other end: Keep forward past the Marks Creek trailhead on Chapmansboro Road, coming directly alongside the Cumberland River. Bridge the Sycamore Creek embayment 3.4 miles from the Marks Creek trailhead and immediately turn right onto the continuation of Chapmansboro Road. Pass several houses and look left for a parking area 0.9 miles from the Sycamore Creek embayment.

The Cumberland River Bicentennial Trail continues west. It is ultimately slated to total 12 miles in length.

CONFEDERATE EARTHWORKS WALK 19

IN BRIEF

This little-used, underrated path at Fort Donelson National Battlefield traverses a corridor of protected land. In addition to running parallel to Confederate earthworks nearly its entire distance, this trail passes over three sizable hills that were artillery batteries connected by these earthworks.

DESCRIPTION

This trail is so little used that it doesn't even have a name. It could be called the Battery Trail, as it passes three Confederate cannon emplacements, or batteries, adjacent to Fort Donelson. It could be called the Earthworks Trail, as it follows alongside Confederate earthworks nearly its entire length. It could be called the Corridor Trail, as it runs easterly along a narrow strip of land that extends like a tail from the main body of the preserved Fort Donelson National Battlefield. And it could be called the Hill Trail, as it starts atop one hill, then alternately dives and climbs two

KEY AT-A-GLANCE INFORMATION

LENGTH: 2.6 miles
CONFIGURATION: There-and-back
DIFFICULTY: Moderate
SCENERY: Forest and field
EXPOSURE: Mostly shady, some sun
TRAFFIC: Very little
TRAIL SURFACE: Grass, leaves
HIKING TIME: 1.7 hours
ACCESS: No fees or permits
MAPS: Available at www.nps.gov/fodo
FACILITIES: Restrooms, water at visitor center

Directions ⟶

From Exit 11 on I-24 northwest of downtown Nashville, take TN 76 3.4 miles west to a traffic light in Clarksville. TN 76 then becomes US 41A north. Keep forward on US 41A north 7.7 miles to US 79. Turn left on US 79 south and follow it 32 miles to reach Fort Donelson National Battlefield, just past the town of Dover, on your right. Stop at the visitor center and obtain a park map. Drive out of the visitor center and turn left on US 79, heading 0.1 mile back toward Dover. Turn right onto an unnamed paved road and follow it a short distance to dead-end at the location of Graves Battery. The trail follows the field downhill as you look toward the cannon at Graves Battery.

GPS Trailhead Coordinates

UTM Zone (WGS84) 16S
Easting 0423160
Northing 4037490
Latitude N 36° 28' 53.5"
Longitude W 87° 51' 27.8"

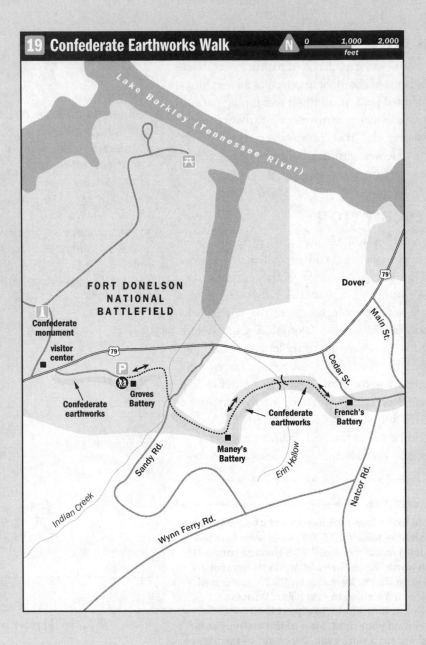

more hills. But the trail shall remain nameless and languish in solitude, while the nearby primary trails of Fort Donelson get more traffic. (See Fort Donelson Battlefield Loop on page 88.)

If you tour Fort Donelson, also take the time to hike this path. It needs some feet on it, and hikers may spot deer as well. Before you hike it, though, stop at the visitor center and get acquainted with the battle that was fought here. Fort Donelson and nearby Fort Henry were built by the Confederate Army to hold sway over the Tennessee and Cumberland rivers, thwarting the Union Army's efforts to use these waterways for troop or supply movements. Fort Henry was poorly located in a low area subject to flooding by the Tennessee River, and in February 1862 was easily bombed into submission by Federal ironclad gunboats. But the Rebels escaped east to Fort Donelson, securely located on a hill with a sweeping view of the Cumberland River. The soldiers of Fort Henry reached Fort Donelson, which was already protected by earthworks, then built an outer perimeter of trenches beyond the fort. These earthworks were stretched along high ground from Hickman Creek in the west to the tiny town of Dover in the east. The earthworks you follow on this hike were part of the outer perimeter.

Federal gunboats couldn't do much against the well-placed Rebel artillery at Fort Donelson, but while the water war was going on Federal troops amassed around the whole Rebel perimeter. The Union crashed the perimeter, but the Rebels pushed them back. In the confusion of battle, the Rebels were ordered to return to their original positions behind the earthworks. The Union attacked again, retaking territory they had lost and gaining some, to boot. Finally, most of the Confederate soldiers escaped southeasterly to Nashville, leaving too few to defend Fort Donelson, which was surrendered to Union General Ulysses S. Grant the next day.

While you're hiking, imagine Confederate and Union troops poised on either side of the earthworks beside you. Leave the circular parking area and head downhill on the grassy part of the corridor. A cannon representing Graves Battery is to your right, and a small brown hiker sign leads the way downhill. The mowed field is cut a little lower along the barely discernible trail. Dive off the hill to reach a wooded flat on your left, and the earthworks will be to your right. Cross a quaint little bridge that passes over a clear stream named Indian Creek. Keep forward beyond the bridge through a field flanked on the left by cedar trees.

Reach Sandy Road and continue forward; an interpretive sign about the activities of Nathan Bedford Forrest stands to your left. Then ascend the wooded hill ahead of you. It is easy to see the narrowness of this protected corridor as houses are visible nearby. Tall cedar and oak trees shade the route, and the earthworks remain to your right. Keep up the steep hill and top out at the location of Maney's Battery. It is easy to see why the Rebel army picked this hilltop with its potential views. Trees were felled back then to open points of observation and clear lines of fire. This four-cannon unit was placed here, along with French's Battery on the next hill, to keep the Union from sneaking down Erin Hollow, where you are headed, and attacking Fort Donelson.

Turn left at Maney's Battery, now descending, again, a long hill. The Rebel trenches remain to your right. Shortly you'll arrive at the bottom of Erin Hollow and span the intermittent stream on a wooden bridge. The trail here becomes a bit obscure. Begin climbing uphill, keeping the earthworks to your right.

The trail opens in a field and climbs steeply to the third hill, on top of which is a most attractive setting. Large hardwoods flank a level grassy area, the site of French's Battery (interpretive signs relate the site's history). Ahead is a small parking area, Cedar Street, and the end of this hike. Retrace your steps through the hills and hollows back to Graves Battery.

NEARBY/RELATED ACTIVITIES

Fort Donelson National Battlefield has an interesting museum, an auto tour, and a nice picnic area. For more information, visit **www.nps.gov/fodo.**

DUNBAR CAVE STATE NATURAL AREA LOOP 20

IN BRIEF

This hike uses two park trails to form a loop. It travels in the woods, along Swan Lake and beside the park's namesake Dunbar Cave. If the walk doesn't do enough for your legs, consider adding a cave tour, which follows underground paths.

DESCRIPTION

Let's face it, Dunbar Cave was preserved more for its underground features than those that the sun shines upon. However, its above-ground features are attractive and as worthy of a visit as the cave. The city of Clarksville has grown around Dunbar Cave State Natural Area, creating a suburban park in the process and making the green space it provides even more valuable. These 110 acres are mostly former farmland, complemented by a lake fed by springs flowing from Dunbar Cave.

Your loop hike traverses the Lake Trail and the Recovery Trail, which is named for the surrounding forest that has recovered from clearing. So strap on your boots and come on up for a hike. Consider a little underground walk too.

Leave the upper parking area and start the Recovery–Short Loop Trail. Picnic tables are scattered around the trailhead. Keep forward,

KEY AT-A-GLANCE INFORMATION

LENGTH: 1.8 miles

CONFIGURATION: Loop

DIFFICULTY: Easy

SCENERY: Hardwood and cedar forest, lake, cave entrance

EXPOSURE: Mostly shady

TRAFFIC: Fairly steady from locals

TRAIL SURFACE: Leaves, dirt, rocks, pavement

HIKING TIME: 1.2 hours

ACCESS: No fees or permits

MAPS: Available at www.tennessee.gov/environment/parks/Dunbar Cave

FACILITIES: Restrooms, water at visitor center

Directions

From Exit 4 on I-24 northwest of downtown Nashville, take US 79 south 4.2 miles to intersect Dunbar Cave Road. Turn left on Dunbar Cave Road and follow it 1.2 miles to Old Dunbar Cave Road. Turn left on Old Dunbar Cave Road and drive just a short distance to the parking-area entrance on your right. The Recovery Trail starts at the upper end of the parking area.

GPS Trailhead Coordinates

UTM Zone (WGS84) 16S

Easting   0472600

Northing 4044840

Latitude   N 36° 33' 1.9"

Longitude W 87° 18' 22.2"

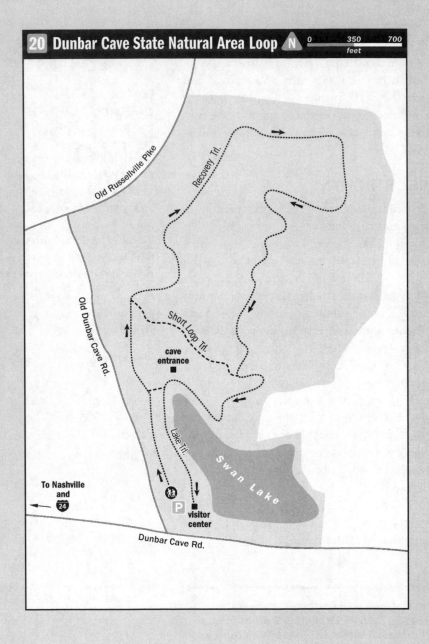

following a former road of crumbling pavement that once led to Dunbar Cave, and you'll see Swan Lake down the hill to your right. At 0.1 mile, a side trail leads right to the entrance of Dunbar Cave. You may not be able to keep your curiosity down, so go ahead and walk to the mouth of the cave. It has a cathedral-like opening, though the actual cave entrance is much smaller. It is easy to visualize live-band music playing in the cave mouth when country-music legend Roy Acuff owned it. He and others not only held concerts and dances here but also broadcast a live country-music radio program from Dunbar. Before that, in the 1880s, the cave and adjacent springs, now used to fill Swan Lake, were parts of a mineral-springs resort. And before that, Tennessee's pre-Columbian Native Americans used it for shelter. Upon the arrival of Tennessee's settlers, a fellow named Dunbar bought the land and gave the cave its name. The state of Tennessee purchased and took over the land and its underground treasures in 1972.

Return to the Recovery Trail (the crumbling pavement has given way to natural trail surface), keep forward, and pass through a cleared area. Just ahead, the Short Loop Trail turns right. The Recovery Trail keeps forward up a hollow and curves right, uphill, through oak woods. Top out in a cedar thicket, drop down the hill, and take the first of three right turns to enter bottomland populated with sycamore trees. The older forest is flanked by a rocky hillside to your right. Wildflowers abound in this bottom during spring.

Ascend away from the bottom to meet the Short Loop at mile 1.2, which comes in from the right. Here, the Recovery Trail once kept forward, but it has since been rerouted to descend toward Swan Lake in a more snakelike, less erosive route. Old Christmas trees have been placed on the former trail route to prevent erosion. Turn left at the junction, following the newer Recovery Trail as it makes its way to Swan Lake. Large oak trees shade the now-paved path along the lake.

The visitor center is visible across the water. This white building was once part of the resort and was converted to park offices and informative displays after being acquired by Tennessee State Parks. Follow the paved path toward the mouth of Dunbar Cave, and you'll reach the columnar concrete addition to the cave mouth; this area may be busy in summer. Beneath you is the spring upwelling that has been flooded by the damming of Swan Lake in 1933. Circle past the cave entrance, still on the lake perimeter. The geese and ducks you'll see here may be looking for handouts because park visitors often feed them. Shortly you'll reach the steps to access the visitor center and the parking area from where you started.

NEARBY/RELATED ACTIVITIES

Dunbar Cave State Natural Area offers cave tours daily during summer, weekends during spring and fall, and at least one weekend per month in winter. Dunbar Cave has 8 miles of explored and surveyed passages that extend about a half mile into the cave, and it maintains a constant 58°F temperature year-round. Groups touring the cave are encouraged to make reservations. Call ahead for exact tour times and fees at (931) 532-0001, or visit **www.tnstateparks.com.**

21 FORT DONELSON BATTLEFIELD LOOP

 KEY AT-A-GLANCE INFORMATION

LENGTH: 3.3 miles

CONFIGURATION: Loop

DIFFICULTY: Moderate

SCENERY: Forests, fields, hardwood ravines, big river

EXPOSURE: Mostly shady

TRAFFIC: Busy on nice weekends and holidays

TRAIL SURFACE: Dirt, mulch, grass

HIKING TIME: 2.5 hours

ACCESS: No fees or permits

MAPS: Available at www.nps.gov/ fodo

FACILITIES: Restrooms, water at visitor center and picnic area

GPS Trailhead Coordinates

UTM Zone (WGS84)   16S

Easting   0422680

Northing   4037550

Latitude   N 36° 28' 55.4"

Longitude   W 87° 51' 46.5"

IN BRIEF

This hike loops the perimeter of Fort Donelson National Battlefield, on the shores of Lake Barkley. Along the way, it visits a monument, river batteries, troop trenches, and log huts from the Civil War. You will be surprised at both the steepness of the terrain and the natural beauty that accompanies this special place.

DESCRIPTION

This is one of Middle Tennessee's great unsung hikes. The historical importance of the trailside location is obvious, but the setting will surprise you. Travel along flanks of Confederate earthworks erected to protect Fort Donelson, which in turn guarded the lower Cumberland River. Pass a tall monument to Confederate soldiers. Then drop to the shores of Lake Barkley to reach Fort Donelson, where river batteries look over a stunning sweep of the Cumberland River. Visit log-hut replicas that housed Confederate troops, and enjoy a woods walk while returning to the visitor center and completing the loop.

To gain an understanding of this battle, which was the first success in the Union's plan to split the Confederacy in two, stop by the

Directions

From Exit 11 on I-24 northwest of downtown Nashville, take TN 76 west 3.4 miles to a traffic light in Clarksville. TN 76 then becomes US 41A north. Keep forward on US 41A north 7.7 miles to US 79. Turn left on US 79 south and follow it 32 miles to reach Fort Donelson National Battlefield, just past the town of Dover, which is on your right. Park at the visitor center. The Donelson Trail starts near the cannon to your left as you look outward from the visitor center.

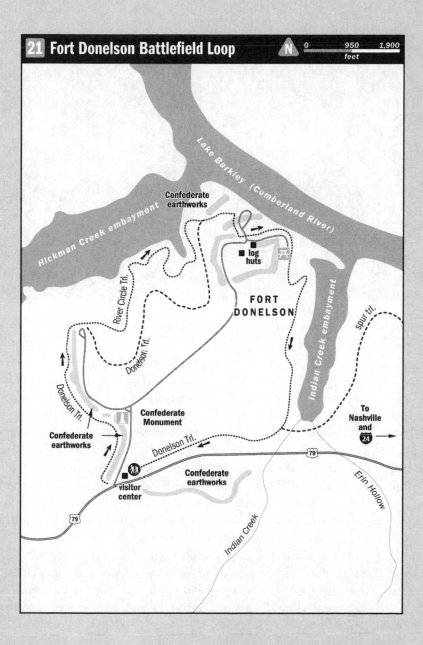

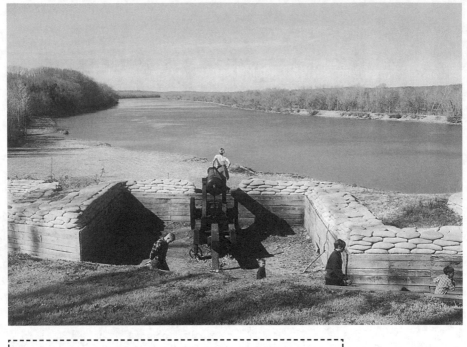

Panoramic sweep of the Cumberland opens at the Upper River Battery.

visitor center and learn more. In summary, the Confederates fled nearby Fort
Henry after being overwhelmed by Union forces. The Union soldiers followed
and began surrounding the Rebels, who had hastily constructed an outer perimeter of earthworks to protect Fort Donelson. Seeing the futility of their own position, the Rebels cleared an escape route up the Cumberland and departed. Others
were left to defend the fort and eventually surrendered to Union General Ulysses
S. Grant. This battle was the first step from obscurity for the general.

The trail begins near the six-pound cannon, where a sign reads "Donelson
Trail, 3.1 miles." In other places the trail is denoted with brown signs that have
hiker symbols on them. Turn right as you face the sign here, and begin walking a
mowed path; Confederate earthworks will be on your right, and the hillside drops
steeply to your left. Basically, the earthworks are trenches that protected soldiers.
Johnny Reb set up these earthworks, using the steep terrain as an added measure
of defense. The Union soldiers had to ascend the hills and storm the trenches to
breach this outer perimeter. The setting is attractive with the mixture of scattered
trees, grass, and woods.

Shortly, you'll reach the Confederate Monument on your right. This tall
stone pillar is fronted with a metal Confederate soldier in uniform. Return to the
trail and keep north along the Rebel trenches, soon passing the site of Union
General C. F. Smith's attack and subsequent capture of the earthworks. Ahead is
the site of Jackson's Battery, a Confederate position later abandoned when the
Rebels decided to break for Nashville.

Reach a trail junction at 0.5 miles. Split left onto the River Circle Trail, which soon dives into the Hickman Creek embayment. Cross and follow an intermittent branch to the embayment. Parallel the embayment, then suddenly climb steeply while circling around a ravine. Come near a field, then turn away and drop to a steeply cut hollow. Cross a footbridge over the tiny stream. Just past the footbridge on the right is a rocked-in spring that may have provided water for soldiers during battle.

Pass along the Hickman Creek embayment once more, before intersecting the Donelson Trail at mile 1.7. Veer left onto the Donelson Trail and soon you'll come out at the Upper River Battery. Here, Confederates used heavy artillery to bombard Union ironclad gunboats into withdrawing. It is easy to see that these well-placed cannons could control the Cumberland River at this point. What you see today is Lake Barkley, formed by the downstream damming of the Cumberland River.

The trail becomes hard to follow at this point. Leave the River batteries and climb uphill on the road toward the log-hut replicas, which are modeled after those that housed Confederate soldiers but were burned down after the Union took over to fight a measles outbreak. Turn left on the road that leads to the Luncheon Area, which is the first picnic area I've ever seen referred to in this way. Anyway, reach the picnic area and look for a huge oak tree backed by earthworks. The trail picks up again here, descending to a ravine along more earthworks (look for a hiker symbol on a small brown sign). The path is mowed as it passes through an open field. Heading south, soon reenter woods and climb to enter a thick pine grove. At mile 2.4, make a sharp left onto an old roadbed. Then pass through low woods before leaving right from the roadbed and climbing to another pine grove.

At mile 2.7, reach a trail junction. Here, the Spur Trail leads left 1.3 miles to the Fort Donelson National Cemetery. The Donelson Trail turns right in south-facing hickory–oak woods, then dives into a ravine. Cross an intermittent streambed on a footbridge, then climb out of the ravine by switchbacks. Shortly reach the backside of the visitor center and complete the loop.

NEARBY/RELATED ACTIVITIES

Fort Donelson National Battlefield has an interesting museum and historical information. The Confederate Earthworks Walk, which is part of Fort Donelson, is also detailed in this book (see page 81). For more information, please visit **www.nps.gov/fodo.**

22 HENRY HOLLOW LOOP

KEY AT-A-GLANCE INFORMATION

LENGTH: 2.1 miles
CONFIGURATION: Loop
DIFFICULTY: Moderate
SCENERY: Streamside woods, ridgetop woods
EXPOSURE: Mostly shaded
TRAFFIC: Busy on weekends
TRAIL SURFACE: Dirt and rocks
HIKING TIME: 1.75 hours
ACCESS: No fees or permits
MAPS: Available at trailside kiosk
FACILITIES: Restroom, picnic tables at parking area

IN BRIEF

This path is the gem of Beaman Park. It shows off the high and the low of this northwest Nashville preserve that has finally been opened to the public. Start along clear Henry Creek and ascend a deeply cut hollow full of wildflowers and other moisture-loving species. The path then heads to the oak-covered ridgetops before returning to the low end of Henry Hollow near Little Marrowbone Creek.

DESCRIPTION

Beaman Park, Nashville's newest big park, is the setting for the Henry Hollow trail, a first-rate spring wildflower destination. If you visited this park once a week starting in late March, you would see new wildflowers—including spring beauties, trillium, phlox, trout lily, toothwort, shooting stars, Jacobs Ladder, dwarf crested iris, and more—blooming every trip. Summer and fall bring their share of flowers too.

This path begins at the Creekside Trailhead of Beaman Park. While here, notice the shortleaf pines around the parking area; these trees are uncommon in Middle Tennessee. Leave the stone gateway trailhead on a gravel

GPS Trailhead Coordinates

UTM Zone (WGS84) 16S
Easting   0508570
Northing 4014010
Latitude   N 36° 16' 22.5"
Longitude W 86° 54' 17.0"

Directions

From Exit 204 on I-40 west of downtown Nashville, take TN 155, Briley Parkway, north to Exit 24, Ashland City, TN 12. Head east on TN 12 south and follow it 0.4 miles to Eaton Creek Road. Turn left on Eaton Creek Road and follow it 5 miles to Little Marrowbone Road. Turn left on Little Marrowbone Road and follow it 0.6 miles to Beaman Park on your left. The Creekside Trailhead is immediately to the left once you enter the park.

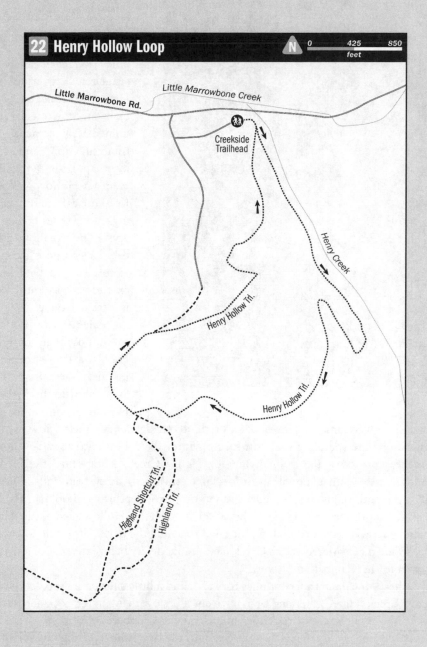

22 Henry Hollow Loop

N

0   425   850
feet

Little Marrowbone Rd.

Little Marrowbone Creek

Creekside
Trailhead

Henry Creek

Henry Hollow Trl.

Henry Hollow Trl.

Highland Shortcut Trl.

Highland Trl.

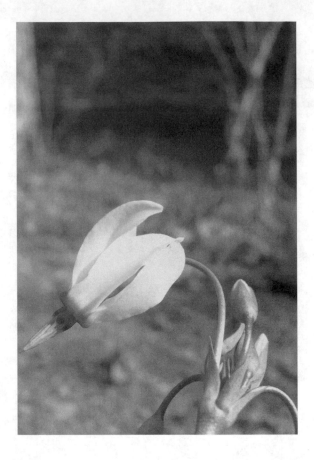

Shooting star is one of many spring wildflowers in Henry Hollow.

path bordered by more pines to reach a stone semicircle overlooking Henry Creek. The path turns up the creek and immediately reaches a trail junction and the loop portion of the Henry Hollow Trail. Keep forward here, heading along the creek, a crystalline stream spilling over layer upon layer of exposed shale that extends across the creek in thin panes. This unspoiled stream is typical of those that drain the Highland Rim surrounding the Nashville Basin. Stay above the creek, passing a contemplation bench. Beech, sycamore, dogwood, and redbuds shade Henry Creek below, which flows in a wide sparkling sheet on sunny winter days. Intermittent wet-weather branches cut across the trail, diving for Henry Creek. After rains, the feeder branches, also with exposed layers of shale, turn into noisy waterfalls. At 0.4 miles, the path spans such a feeder branch on a wooden bridge. Look across the creek for more feeder branches. The streams of Henry Hollow feed Little Marrowbone Creek, which runs along the road reaching the park. Little Marrowbone Creek then meets Marrowbone Creek near Ashland City before the pair of streams flows into the Cumberland River.

Ahead, the main trail continues forward, and a little spur path veers left along Henry Creek. Here, water and time have cut a big overhang in the rock across the creek, one reminiscent of rock formations on the Cumberland Plateau. A feeder branch cuts into Henry Creek just upstream of the overhang, creating low stairstep cascades on Henry Creek. The creek gathers in shallow pools where minnows dart away as you near them. Look in the water for crawdads, too, with their pincers ready to capture prey. Kids could have a blast playing in Henry Creek.

At 0.5 miles, the white-blazed trail leaves Henry Creek and turns up the hillside to your right, using a pair of switchbacks to ease the grade. Watch for more wildflowers as the trail works up this steep slope to make a four-way trail junction at 1.3 miles. You are now in oak woods. Here, Highland Trail goes off to the left, and Highland Shortcut Trail continues forward. To the right, the Henry Hollow and Highland trails run in conjunction with one another to reach a second junction at 1.5 miles; you'll see the Highland Trailhead at this second junction.

The Henry Hollow Trail curves off the ridgetop, working along an oak-dominated south-facing slope. The open woods are completely different here compared with the lush creekside forest. The trail continues easing into Henry Hollow, eventually returning to bottomland and reaching a trail junction at 2 miles. From here, retrace your steps back to the trailhead.

NEARBY/RELATED ACTIVITIES

Guided hikes and other programs are periodically held at Beaman Park. Check the park kiosk or **www.nashville.gov/parks** for more information. The Highland Trail is also located at Beaman Park and is detailed in this guidebook (see page 100).

23 HIDDEN LAKE DOUBLE LOOP

KEY AT-A-GLANCE INFORMATION

LENGTH: 1.6 miles

CONFIGURATION: Double loop

DIFFICULTY: Easy to moderate

SCENERY: Rock bluffs, old quarry, cedar forest

EXPOSURE: Mostly shady

TRAFFIC: Moderate on weekends

TRAIL SURFACE: Grass, rocks, dirt, leaves

HIKING TIME: 1 hour

ACCESS: No fees or permits

MAPS: Available at www.tennessee .gov/environment/parks/Harpeth River/images/parkmap.pdf

FACILITIES: None

IN BRIEF

This hike takes place on a recently acquired tract of Harpeth River State Park. It travels through transitioning fields before entering woodland to reach bluffs above the Harpeth River. The trail then straddles the bluffs with the Harpeth on one side and Hidden Lake on the other before looping around a wooded knob past a tourist resort.

DESCRIPTION

Leave the open gravel parking area and enter a field to follow a grassy track toward Hidden Lake. A separate route heads downhill toward Harpeth River and is a canoe-kayak access point. Travel northwest through open terrain scattered with bird boxes. This former pasture is being managed for songbirds. The Harpeth River flows to your left beyond the screen of trees in the lower floodplain. At 0.2 miles, you'll reach a trail junction. Here, the Bluebird Loop heads right through the field. This will be your return route. For now, keep straight into the woodland, ambling on an old roadbed beside a small creek to your left. This up-and-coming forest is favorable for birds. It offers a mixture of young trees, bushes, and waterside habitat that all make for a rich ecosystem—the more habitat variety, the more

GPS Trailhead Coordinates

UTM Zone (WGS84) 16S

Easting   0497790

Northing   3993698

Latitude   N 36° 5' 16.38"

Longitude   W 87° 1' 28.31"

Directions

From Exit 192 on I-40, take McCrory Lane north 0.9 miles, crossing the Harpeth River, then immediately look left for the trailhead parking area.

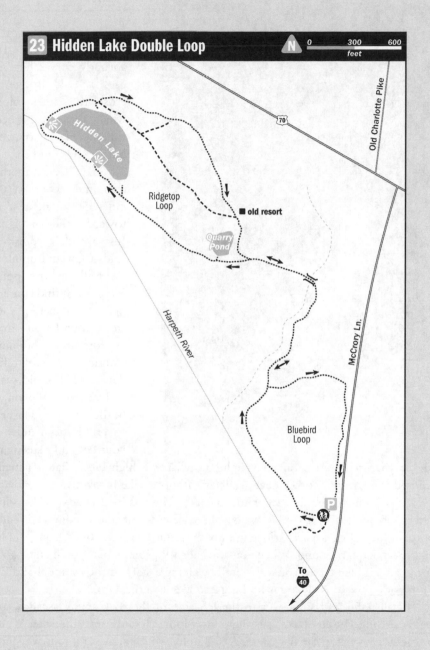

23 Hidden Lake Double Loop

N

0   300   600
feet

Old Charlotte Pike

70

Hidden Lake

Ridgetop
Loop

■ old resort

Quarry
Pond

Harpeth River

McCrory Ln.

Bluebird
Loop

P

To
40

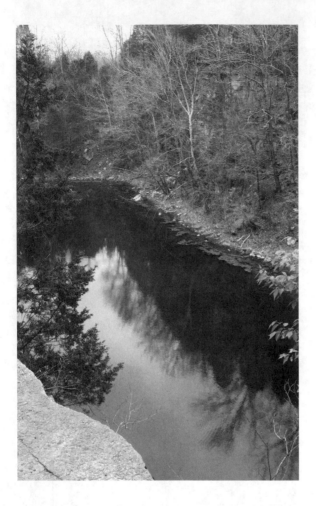

View of Hidden Lake from a bluff

species that can enjoy it. At 0.4 miles, the trail abruptly curves left and uses an old bridge to cross the creek along which you've been walking. Hackberry trees border the trail here.

You'll reach another trail intersection at 0.5 miles. Stay left, heading toward Hidden Lake. Just ahead, a spur trail leads right and uphill to a small quarry pond. Here you'll find contemplation benches and stone foundations from a forgotten building. Continue toward Hidden Lake. The old roadbed you are following is bordered by Harpeth River bottomland on your left and a steep hillside to your right. Also on your right, watch for a high bluff that is actually exposed stone from another quarry, albeit without a lake below it.

At 0.7 miles, you'll reach Hidden Lake. The roadbed heads to the silent waters surrounded by cut-rock walls. The trail cuts left and becomes a slender footpath ascending a rocky ridgeline dividing the Harpeth River from Hidden Lake, a large quarry pond. When you reach a rock prominence, you'll enjoy good views into Hidden Lake. You are literally walking a stacked rock spine that drops off in both directions. There is nothing else like it in this book.

Finally, the trail slips over to the left side of the rock spine, ascends, and begins circling Hidden Lake, passing a vista looking south into the lake. Watch for cactus growing in the dry rocks. At 0.8 miles, you'll arrive at a four-way junction. To your far right, stone steps lead to the water's edge. To your right, a trail shortcuts the loop. Keep straight to make the longest loop possible and trace a roadbed to another junction at 0.9 miles. Again, continue heading straight to reach yet another junction at 1.1 miles. Check out the remains of an old 1940s resort; if you peer through the woods to your right, the quarry pond lies below. An examination of the building reveals no pioneer cabin but rather a "newer" old place. The structure itself is concrete block covered with finishing concrete on the outside. A water tank, electrical hookups, and more reveal the modernity of the structure. Look for the basketball rim around which an ancient cedar tree has grown. Shortly, you'll complete Ridgetop Loop and begin backtracking toward the trailhead. At 1.4 miles, you'll reach the Bluebird Loop. Turn left here, meandering through the field near McCrory Lane before completing the loop at 1.6 miles.

NEARBY/RELATED ACTIVITIES

The Hidden Lake Tract of Harpeth River State Park also has a canoe launch, and the Harpeth River is ready and available for floating. You can also visit the Newsom's Mill Tract of Harpeth River State Park. For more information, visit **www .tennessee.gov/environment/parks/HarpethRiver.**

24 HIGHLAND TRAIL AT BEAMAN PARK

KEY AT-A-GLANCE INFORMATION

LENGTH: 4.2 miles

CONFIGURATION: Out-and-back

DIFFICULTY: Moderate

SCENERY: Ridgetop woodlands

EXPOSURE: Mostly shady

TRAFFIC: Moderate to busy on weekends

TRAIL SURFACE: Dirt

HIKING TIME: 2 hours

ACCESS: No fees or permits

MAPS: Available at trailside kiosk

FACILITIES: Restroom, picnic tables at parking area

IN BRIEF

This ridge-running trail at Beaman Park winds through Highland Rim woodlands to end among big oaks. Never too steep, the path nevertheless offers views into incredibly precipitous hollows that cut deep into the Highland Rim.

DESCRIPTION

The Highland Trail at Beaman Park was a long time in the making. The 1,500-acre tract was purchased by the city of Nashville in 1996, and it took nearly ten years from the time of purchase until the park was open for unsupervised visitation as it is today. The Highland Trail will show you that this part of Davidson County is rugged, steep, and still a little wild. It also will show you that Alvin Beaman, a former member of the city park board, would be proud of his wife's donation of the money to buy this slice of the Highland Rim. You will appreciate the group of doctors who sold the tract to the state at half its appraised value. This land, known to early Nashvillians as Paradise Ridge, for brothers named Paradise, is now a natural paradise where clear streams have cut surprisingly steep hollows divided by narrow ridges of hickory and oak, places where deer and turkey roam.

GPS Trailhead Coordinates

UTM Zone (WGS84) 16S

Easting   0508510

Northing   4013220

Latitude   N 36° 15' 56.5"

Longitude W 86° 54' 18.7"

Directions

From Exit 204 on I-40 west of downtown Nashville, take TN 155, Briley Parkway, north to Exit 24, Ashland City, TN 12. Head east on TN 12 south and follow it 0.4 miles to Eaton Creek Road. Turn left on Eaton Creek Road and follow it 5 miles to Little Marrowbone Road. Turn left on Little Marrowbone Road and follow it 0.6 miles to Beaman Park on your left. The Highland Trailhead is up the hill once you enter the park.

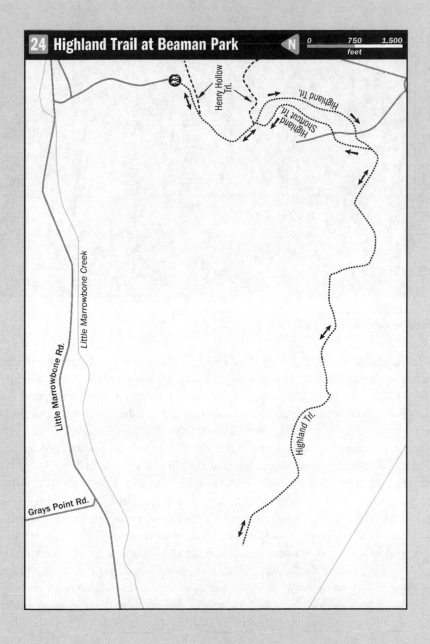

24 Highland Trail at Beaman Park

N

0   750   1,500
feet

Henry Hollow Trl.

Highland Trl.

Highland Shortcut Trl

Little Marrowbone Creek

Little Marrowbone Rd.

Highland Trl.

Grays Point Rd.

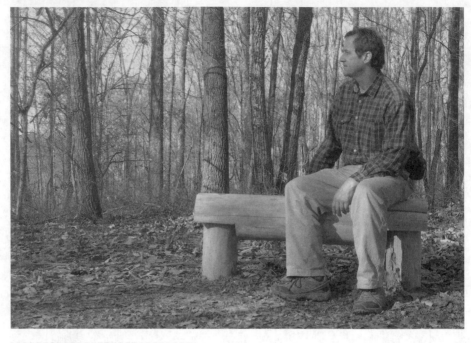

Author relaxing on bench at trail's end

The park has been tastefully developed, as you will see at the trailhead where a stone entryway and kiosk serve as your corridor to the hike. The Highland Trail, true to its name, stays on the highest of ridges, meandering amid oaks aplenty. Descend from the trailhead to join an old roadbed, and meet one end of the Henry Hollow Trail. Stay forward with the red-blazed Highland Trail as it drifts over to the south side of the ridge, skirting a deep hollow to your left.

The wide track soon reaches another trail junction: to your left, Henry Hollow Trail leads to Henry Creek; Highland Trail Shortcut goes off to the right. You will use the shortcut on your return. Continue forward, staying on the Highland Trail. The dirt-and-rock track runs south amid young forest. At 0.6 miles, you'll reach old Blueberry Hill Road, a service road that goes off to the left. Blueberry Hill is yet another name this area had when it was a private hunting preserve. The Highland Trail keeps right. The young trees here reveal another use this land had—timber extraction. You are now on an old logging road.

In spring, look for bluets and pussy toes, wildflowers that can grow in drier places such as this hickory–oak forest. Reach the other end of the Highland Shortcut Trail in a gap at 0.8 miles. Look around here, and notice that on either side of you the land drops off precipitously. The trail climbs away from the gap in an area of many tulip trees. These trees often are the first to regenerate after an area has been cleared, as this ridge undoubtedly once was. By 1.3 miles, the canopy is often open overhead, a result of relic clearings that haven't completely reforested.

Also notice the preponderance of briers rising in tangles from the forest floor and merging with younger trees. These areas allow views of the adjacent ridges divided by chasmlike streamsheds.

The Highland Trail continues a pattern of undulating between narrow gaps and knobs, heading west into more mature woods. At 2.1 miles, the trail ends at a level knob. Contemplation benches allow hikers to rest and relax while enjoying this reward. They can also contemplate hiking back 2.1 miles to the trailhead. On the return trip, try to see what you may have missed on the way in. Also, hikers should take the Highland Shortcut Trail while returning. The twisting, winding singletrack footpath actually isn't any shorter, but it covers new terrain and works around the edges of deep hollows. It also travels through moister woods, which offer more wildflowers in spring.

NEARBY/RELATED ACTIVITIES

Guided hikes and other programs are periodically held at Beaman Park. Check the park kiosk or **www.nashville.gov/parks** for more information. The Henry Hollow Loop is also located at Beaman Park and is detailed in this guidebook (see page 92).

25 JOHNSONVILLE STATE HISTORIC AREA LOOP

KEY AT-A-GLANCE INFORMATION

LENGTH: 2.6 miles

CONFIGURATION: Loop

DIFFICULTY: Easy to moderate

SCENERY: Hardwood forest, huge lake

EXPOSURE: Mostly shady

TRAFFIC: Not much

TRAIL SURFACE: Leaves, dirt, rocks, a little pavement

HIKING TIME: 1.8 hours

ACCESS: No fees or permits

MAPS: Johnsonville State Historic Area (SHA) Trails Map, available at kiosk at park entrance

FACILITIES: Restrooms, water at picnic area

SPECIAL COMMENTS: This is one of many loop possibilities here.

GPS Trailhead Coordinates

UTM Zone (WGS84)　16S

Easting　0413000

Northing　3991090

Latitude　N 36° 3' 44.6"

Longitude　W 86° 57' 56.8"

IN BRIEF

Set along the banks of the Tennessee River, this hike loops through an area that was once a town, a railroad, and a Civil War battle site. Now dammed as Kentucky Lake, the hilly terrain along the lake provides an attractive setting for this walk into Tennessee history.

DESCRIPTION

Just a minor steamboat landing before the Civil War, the landing at Johnsonville was taken over by the Union and converted to a river-rail transfer point. During this time, the Union had also built a railroad connecting this landing to Nashville, enabling movement of supplies from the North by water and land. By train from Johnsonville, supplies were delivered to Nashville and south to Atlanta, where Sherman was preparing his ruthless "March to the Sea."

Things looked grim for the Rebels. Their best chance was to cut off Union supplies and force the Union soldiers to retreat from Georgia to keep a safe supply line. Tennessee's General Nathan Bedford Forrest decided to

----

Directions ─────────────────────────────→

From Exit 172 on I-40 west of Nashville, take TN 46 north 4.4 miles to US 70 Business west near Dickson. Stay on US 70 Business west 1.3 miles to US 70 west. Turn left and stay on US 70 west 33 miles to Nell Beard Road. Turn right on Nell Beard Road and follow it 2.3 miles to Old Johnsonville Road. Turn left on Old Johnsonville Road and follow it 0.3 miles to the park entrance. Pick up a trail map at the entrance, continue forward 0.3 miles on the paved road, and park at the back of the lower picnic area. The hike starts on the narrow paved trail at the rear of the parking area.

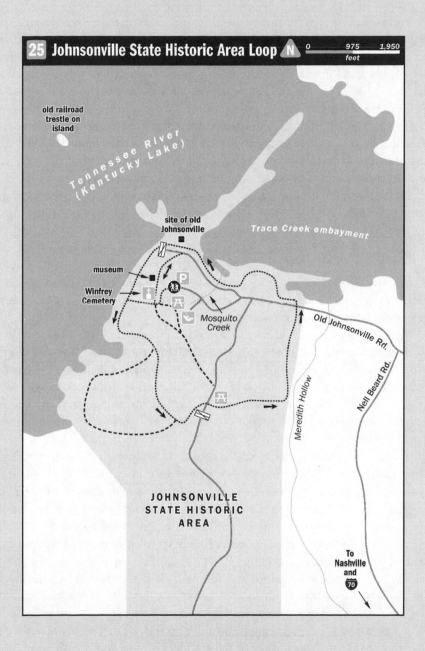

25 Johnsonville State Historic Area Loop

old railroad trestle on island

Tennessee River (Kentucky Lake)

site of old Johnsonville

Trace Creek embayment

museum

Winfrey Cemetery

Mosquito Creek

Old Johnsonville Rd.

Meredith Hollow

Nell Beard Rd.

JOHNSONVILLE STATE HISTORIC AREA

To Nashville and 70

0   975   1,950
feet

attack and take Johnsonville to cut off the supply route and turn the South's sinking fortunes of war.

Forrest came north from Paris Landing on the Tennessee River, having captured a couple of Union boats; other cavalry members came by land. The general
set up cannons at Pilot Knob, across the river from Johnsonville. On November
4, 1864, his small forces annihilated the Union's naval forces around Johnsonville, destroying 3 gunboats, 11 transports, 18 barges, and millions of dollars
worth of Union supplies.

This is the only time in recorded history that men on horses engaged and
defeated a naval force. The engagement was a success for the South, but Sherman
completed his March to the Sea, seizing supplies from citizens along the way. This
march split the South in two and essentially ended the Civil War.

In 1945, the Tennessee Valley Authority bought the land for the damming
of Kentucky Lake, and Johnsonville was abandoned. The railroad was rerouted
after the river damming.

Today, the area is a state park with hiking trails you can enjoy. The trail
system at Johnsonville State Historic Area adds up to 6 miles. At least that's what
the park brochure states. You may have to make a few loops and double back on
yourself to get all the miles in, but so what? Take your time looking around for
clues of old homesites and signs of the town.

Start this loop at the back of the lower picnic area. Look for a narrow paved
trail crossing a small culvert and ascending a hill into the woods. This path shortly
crosses a paved road. Ahead of you is the park museum, which may or may not
be open. It's worth a look if it's open; if it's not, turn left to check out the Winfrey Cemetery. Oddly, the internment is situated inside the earthen defenses
(redoubt) atop this hill. This redoubt was placed here to protect the rail and transfer point from the Rebels.

To your left are the paved parking area and the Russ Manning Nature Trail.
Do not take this path. Rather, as you are facing the trail sign, look to the right for
a path entering young brush and woods; it is marked with a small wooden sign
that reads "Trail." These signs are placed along the path to keep you headed the
right way. Follow this trail as it precipitously dives to an old roadbed paralleling
the Tennessee River, now impounded as Kentucky Lake. Remember this point, as
it will be part of your return route.

Turn left on the old roadbed and follow it along the river. The path shortly
goes to the left from the roadbed and traverses a flat area of big hickories and
oaks. Circle around the flat, crossing intermittent streambeds, to make a second
trail junction at 0.7 miles. Turn left, heading up the hill that climbs steeply, and
reach a contemplation bench where the trail levels off. Continue forward, ram-
bling through the woods to reach another trail junction at mile 1. Turn left here,
and shortly reach the end of a paved turnaround at the other park picnic area.

Cross the paved road, passing near a children's swing. The trail then dives
into Meredith Hollow, where a clear stream makes a torturous course through

the formerly settled flat. Daffodils abound in early March. Note that this area can be mucky.

Continue following the trail down Meredith Hollow to reach the park entrance road. Turn left, walk a short distance, and look for a trail entering the woods to your right. Keep forward in this marshy area and reach the raised rail bed fought over by Forrest and the Union. Trace the railroad grade left, as you circle a little knob to your left. Leave the rail bed near some stoneworks and emerge onto a dirt road, where you'll turn right.

The Trace Creek embayment is to your right. Pass the site of a railroad turntable on your left in the marsh of Mosquito Creek. Soon a paved road turns to the left up to the museum. Keep forward to reach the Johnsonville town site. Ahead, the raised rail bed leads into the Tennessee River.

After looking around, continue on the roadbed past a metal gate. A steep hill, where the redoubt and museum are, stands to your left. Kentucky Lake is to your right. The high point across the water, with a building atop it, is Pilot Knob. Continue forward and look for the trail leading left up to the redoubt (you came down this one). Climb the hill, pass the Winfrey Cemetery on your left, and pick up the narrow paved path down to your car and the lower picnic area.

26 MONTGOMERY BELL NORTHEAST LOOP

KEY AT-A-GLANCE INFORMATION

LENGTH: 6 miles

CONFIGURATION: Loop

DIFFICULTY: Moderate

SCENERY: Hardwood forest, creeks, lake

EXPOSURE: Mostly shady

TRAFFIC: Some on weekends

TRAIL SURFACE: Leaves, dirt, rocks

HIKING TIME: 3 hours

ACCESS: No fees or permits required

MAPS: Montgomery Bell Trail Map available at park office

FACILITIES: Water, picnic tables, restroom at park office

GPS Trailhead Coordinates

UTM Zone (WGS84)   16S

Easting   0474520

Northing   3995020

Latitude   N 36° 6' 4.4"

Longitude   W 87° 16' 59.1"

IN BRIEF

This loop traverses varied terrain, showing off the natural beauty Montgomery Bell State Park has to offer. It passes through rich hickory–oak woods, along clear streams, over ridges, and beside a lake. You can enjoy this hike in all seasons.

DESCRIPTION

This is one of those hikes you don't mind doing more than once. It offers variety along the trail, and that variety will change with each season. I have found both the northeastern and southwestern loops of the Montgomery Bell (MB) Trail enjoyable at all times of the year. So pick a day and hit the trail.

Start the northeastern loop from the park office. Walk back toward the park entrance on the main park road, crossing Wildcat Creek on the road bridge. Shortly reach the old park headquarters building on your right. Pick up the MB Trail just beyond the building. Scramble up the hillside, then pick up an old woods road. Begin a moderate but steady ascent through an oak–hickory forest on a narrow singletrack path. An observant eye will notice the older trees that bordered the old road. These contrast with the relatively younger trees growing on the old roadbed.

Pass near a pair of steep, deep hollows on your right before making a hard right at mile

Directions

From Exit 182 on I-40 west of Nashville, head west on TN 96 11 miles to US 70 near Dickson. Turn right on US 70, then head 4 miles east to the state-park entrance, which will be on the right. Enter and park at the office on your right. The loop begins on the main park road near the old park headquarters.

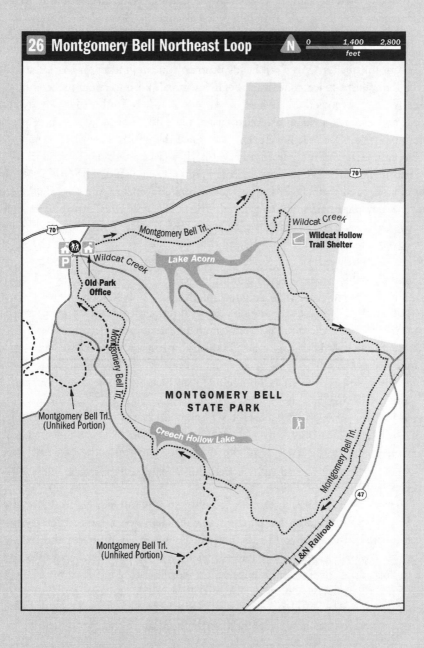

26 Montgomery Bell Northeast Loop

N

0   1,400   2,800
feet

70

Montgomery Bell Trl.

Wildcat Creek

Wildcat Hollow
Trail Shelter

70

Wildcat Creek

Lake Acorn

Old Park
Office

P

Montgomery Bell Trl.

MONTGOMERY BELL
STATE PARK

Montgomery Bell Trl.
(Unhiked Portion)

Creech Hollow Lake

Montgomery Bell Trl.

47

Montgomery Bell Trl.
(Unhiked Portion)

L&N Railroad

1. Begin working your way down toward Wildcat Hollow, passing a small feeder branch, then reaching Wildcat Creek. Descend along Wildcat Creek and arrive at a large feeder stream at mile 1.4. Step over this stream. Dead ahead, up the hill, is the Wildcat Hollow trail shelter, used by backpackers for overnight camping trips. It overlooks the confluence of Wildcat Creek and its unnamed feeder branch.

From the shelter, MB Trail heads upstream in the hollow of the large feeder branch, crossing it twice. The creek begins to break up into small feeder branches of its own as it ascends the lush hollow. At mile 2.1, MB Trail turns away from the hollow and ascends a ridge as it stays inside park boundaries. The concrete park-boundary markers you see have been there since the park's inception in the 1930s.

At mile 2.5, you'll come to a gravel park-service road. Turn left and follow the road toward TN 47, just beyond the gate you see ahead. The MB Trail turns right before reaching the gate and reenters woodland on a newer road that's sometimes used by park personnel to maintain the park's golf course, off to the right.

The walking is easy among the pines and cedars that grow alongside the ever-present oaks. Side trails leave to the right, toward the golf course. At mile 3.5, the MB Trail abruptly leaves the roadbed and turns right into a hollow; this turn is signed and hard to miss. Descend along this hollow, which, with the help of a few other small streams, eventually gathers enough water to feed Creech Hollow Lake. The MB Trail stays along the edge of the hollow before descending to cross the stream that flows through the hollow. Climb away from the stream to reach a trail junction at mile 4.1. Then turn right, as the outer loop of the MB Trail goes to the left and circles the entire park. This other section of the MB Trail is part of the Montgomery Bell Southwest Loop, included in this guidebook (see next page).

The cutoff MB Trail now runs with the orange-blazed Creech Hollow Trail. Descend to the shores of Creech Hollow Lake and skirt the lake's edge in young woods to reach a clearing near the dam. Walk along the lake through the clearing and enter forest on the left side of the lake dam. Drop into the heart of Creech Hollow far below the lake level. A steep bluff flanks the trail, enabling you to grab views of the stream below.

Turn away from Creech Hollow, climbing a ridge to make a trail junction at mile 5.4. Then turn right at the junction, leaving the Creech Hollow Trail behind. Continue along the hardwood ridgeline before reaching a part of the park that looks like it was dug out at one time—it was. Take the wooden steps into an old rock quarry, now covered in pine trees. The stonework you see around the park came from this quarry. Continue forward beyond the quarry, and you'll soon reach a trail junction. Look across the park road for the park office, returning to where you left your vehicle, to complete the loop after 6 miles.

NEARBY/RELATED ACTIVITIES

Montgomery Bell offers a good campground, fishing lakes, picnic areas, an inn, a restaurant, and a golf course. For more information, call (615) 797-9052 or visit **www.tnstateparks.com.**

MONTGOMERY BELL SOUTHWEST LOOP 27

IN BRIEF

This hike explores southwestern Montgomery Bell State Park, making a long loop. First, tread among old pits from an 1800s iron-ore mine. Then pass a historic cabin site where a church denomination was founded and a local cemetery is still in use. Next you'll see the natural beauty at Hall Spring, Lake Woodhaven, and Creech Hollow Lake.

DESCRIPTION

This loop hike is good for those who really want to get out in the woods. The terrain is never difficult, and plenty of places beckon hikers to stop, linger, and contemplate nature and history. Pack some lunch or snacks and make a full day of it. Start the hike on the Montgomery Bell Trail (MB Trail), which leaves the Church Hollow Picnic Area and crosses the road on which you came. The MB Trail is blazed in white, and the Ore Pit Trail is blazed in red. These trails run together for the first and very last portion of the hike.

Head up a hill into a forest of oak, maple, and tulip trees on an old wagon road. You'll reach a trail junction at 0.2 miles and will immediately notice many holes in the ground. These holes, now rounded with time and

KEY AT-A-GLANCE INFORMATION

LENGTH: 6.9 miles
CONFIGURATION: Loop
DIFFICULTY: Moderate
SCENERY: Woods, creeks, lakes
EXPOSURE: Nearly all shady
TRAFFIC: Moderate
TRAIL SURFACE: Dirt, rocks, leaves
HIKING TIME: 4 hours
ACCESS: No fees or permits required
MAPS: Montgomery Bell Trail Map available at park office
FACILITIES: Water at picnic area; picnic tables, restroom at park office

Directions

From Exit 182 on I-40 west of Nashville, head west on TN 96 11 miles to US 70 near Dickson. Turn right on US 70, then head 4 miles east to the state-park entrance, which will be on the right. Enter the park and drive 0.5 miles to a fork in the road by a ball field. Take the right fork, drive forward just a short distance, then take the next right toward Church Hollow. Park in the picnic area, which will be on your left.

GPS Trailhead Coordinates

UTM Zone (WGS84) 16S
Easting   0474060
Northing 3994100
Latitude   N 36° 5' 34.9"
Longitude W 87° 17' 16.1"

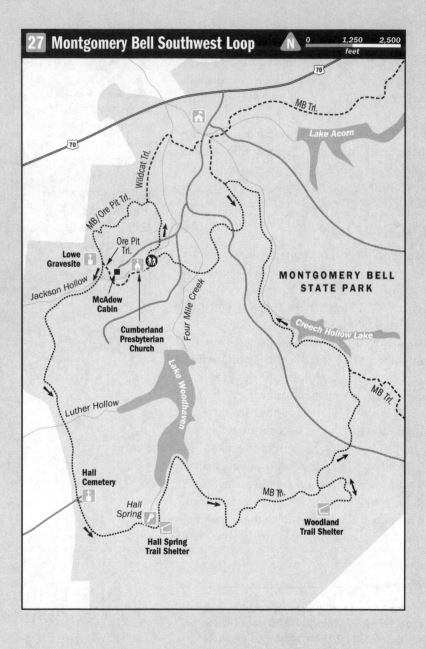

27 Montgomery Bell Southwest Loop

N

0   1,250   2,500
feet

70

MB Trl.

Lake Acorn

70

Wildcat Trl.

MB/Ore Pit Trl.

Ore Pit Trl.

Lowe Gravesite

Jackson Hollow

McAdow Cabin

MONTGOMERY BELL STATE PARK

Creech Hollow Lake

Cumberland Presbyterian Church

Four Mile Creek

MB Trl.

Lake Woodhaven

Luther Hollow

Hall Cemetery

Hall Spring

MB Trl.

Woodland Trail Shelter

Hall Spring Trail Shelter

grown over with trees, are the remains of pits that were dug to extract the area's iron ore, which was fed into Laurel Furnace, located near the picnic area. Trees were cut and turned into charcoal to heat the ore, and water power was used to run a large bellows that blew oxygen into the fire. The molten iron was poured into molds known as "sows," giving rise to the name "pig iron." The discarded leftover material was slag. Most of these furnaces operated 24 hours a day, seven days a week. Can you imagine the heat of these furnaces in summer?

The MB Trail turns left at the junction. This path and park were named for Tennessee's premier iron industrialist of the early 1800s, Montgomery Bell. He established furnaces all over the area. Look around as the path winds between these old pits. The woods, dotted with tall white oaks, display the enduring healing powers of nature. Head downhill and reach a trail junction at mile 1. Here, a side trail leads 75 yards up an old wagon road to the lone grave of Dorothy Lowe, daughter of Sam and Jo Lowe. The girl lived just two years in the early 1900s. After the iron furnaces went cold, the Lowe family most likely farmed this area.

The MB Trail continues downhill and soon reaches a clearing and a cabin. This cabin is a replica of the one in which Sam McAdow, a founder of the Cumberland Presbyterian Church, lived. Back in 1810, religious fervor swept rural areas of the country, and doctrinal differences led McAdow and others to form their own denomination. This cabin has two rooms separated by a "dogtrot," which helped keep the cabin cooler in summer by allowing plenty of shade and dividing the kitchen, with its constant cooking fires, from the bedroom. Notice the giant sugar maples circling the cabin. Just down the field is a chapel that holds services on summer weekends.

The MB Trail passes beyond the cabin and over a clear stream on a footbridge. Look to the left just beyond the bridge at McAdow Spring. The squared-off stones still remain from days when the McAdows drew water from this source. Keep upstream on the creek that forms Jackson Hollow, leaving the Ore Pit Trail behind. Soon pass a concrete marker placed here by the National Park Service, which used this park as a recreation-demonstration project before it was handed over to the state of Tennessee. The MB Trail narrows and rises above the creek and swings around a fern-cloaked hill before leaving Jackson Hollow up a wagon road on a side branch.

Top out on a hill at mile 1.8, and find a resting bench. Descend along the park border to lushly vegetated Luther Hollow, crossing a clear stream on a footbridge with handrails. Climb sharply from Luther Hollow and level out to reach a gravel road at mile 2.5. To your left are a cedar-studded field and the Hall Cemetery, which is still used by local residents. Cross the gravel road, passing around a metal gate, to pick up an old woods road flanked by cedar and dogwood. Drop into a hardwood flat, crossing an often-dry streambed on a footbridge, before reaching the Hall Spring trail shelter; backpackers use this site. Hall Spring is below the shelter and sends forth an estimated 1,000 gallons of

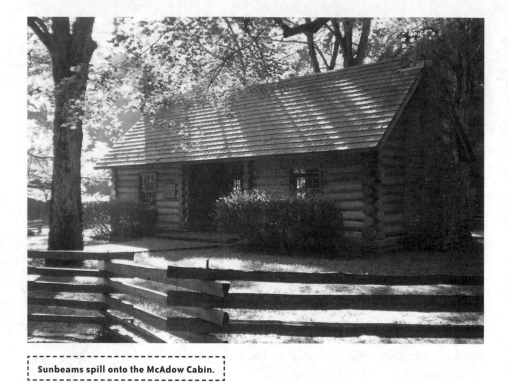

Sunbeams spill onto the McAdow Cabin.

water per minute from a large circular pool. The coolness and clarity of the water are indisputable.

Climb away from the trail shelter and turn north, following translucent Hall Creek past a closed wetland walkway, to reach the shores of the clear Lake Wood-haven, one of three impoundments that dot the state park. Follow the Hall Creek arm of the lake to a vista point and enjoy the view before turning away from the stream along a branch feeding the lake. Eventually, step over this branch and traverse a piney ridgeline. Drop into another drainage and small stream crossing, then make a trail junction at mile 4.2. Here, a side trail leads right for a ten-minute walk to the Woodland trail shelter, another backpacker's campsite set on a hill above a rock-enclosed spring. Occasional yellow signs note that the land adjacent to the trail is being preserved as a Tennessee Natural Area.

The MB Trail climbs through hickory–oak woods to reach a park road at mile 4.5. Keep forward, reaching a trail junction at mile 4.8. Turn left here, as the outer loop of the MB Trail turns to the right and circles the entire park. The cutoff MB Trail now runs with the orange-blazed Creech Hollow Trail. Descend to reach the shores of Creech Hollow Lake, and skirt the lake's edge to reach a clearing near the dam. Continue along the lake through the clearing and enter the woods on the left side of the lake dam. Then drop into the heart of Creech Hol-low far below lake level. A steep bluff flanks the trail.

Turn away from Creech Hollow, climbing a ridge, to make a trail junction at mile 6.1. Turn left here, leaving the Creech Hollow Trail behind. The MB trail, which runs along the ridge before crossing a park road, undulates steeply across two dry ravines before making the most precipitous descent of the hike to reach Four Mile Creek. Span the creek on a footbridge, then head downstream. Note the bluffs across the glassy watercourse. Turn away from the creek, passing a maintenance area and backpacker parking area. Climb into maple–cedar woods before crossing a paved road leading to Lake Woodhaven. You'll enter a full-blown cedar forest before intersecting the Ore Pit Trail again at mile 6.8. Turn right here and descend, bridging a small stream, to enter the Church Hollow picnic area and complete the loop.

NEARBY/RELATED ACTIVITIES

Montgomery Bell has recreation beyond its trail system. It offers a good campground, fishing lakes, picnic areas, an inn, a restaurant, and a golf course. You could incorporate any of the above with a hike. For more information, call (615) 797-9052 or visit **www.tnstateparks.com.**

28 NARROWS OF HARPETH HIKE

KEY AT-A-GLANCE INFORMATION

LENGTH: 1.8 miles

CONFIGURATION: There-and-back

DIFFICULTY: Easy

SCENERY: River, rock bluff, forest

EXPOSURE: Mostly shady

TRAFFIC: Busy on weekends

TRAIL SURFACE: Dirt, rocks

HIKING TIME: 1.3 hours

ACCESS: No fees or permits

MAPS: None available

FACILITIES: Picnic tables

SPECIAL COMMENTS: This trail forks and has two there-and-backs; the 1.8 miles include both there-and-backs.

IN BRIEF

This hike travels along the Harpeth River, passing through an area known as the Narrows. Here, the Harpeth River, in a 5-mile-long bend, nearly curves back on itself. Highlights include a man-made tunnel that cuts across the bend in the river and panoramic views of the Harpeth River and the surrounding countryside.

DESCRIPTION

This State Historic Area, a lesser-known gem of the Tennessee state-park system, is now part of the greater Harpeth River State Park. Today, visitors can float the Harpeth River, picnic and fish on its banks, and hike its trails. Back in the early 1800s, as Montgomery Bell developed the iron-ore industry in Middle Tennessee, he searched for a place to build a water-powered mill on the banks of the Harpeth River. Bell noticed the location where the river made such a bend that it nearly doubled back on itself, separated only by slender but steep bluff. What took one person in a boat 5 miles by water took another on foot a half hour to clamber over. In those 5 miles, the Harpeth dropped several feet. It was here that Bell saw the chance to harness waterpower for

GPS Trailhead Coordinates

UTM Zone (WGS84) 16S

Easting   0489270

Northing   4000570

Latitude   N 36° 9' 6.7"

Longitude   W 87° 7' 8.8"

Directions

From Exit 188 on I-40 west of Nashville, take TN 249 and follow it 2.3 miles to a T intersection with US 70. Turn left, heading west on US 70 2.3 miles to Cedar Hill Road. Turn right on Cedar Hill Road and follow it 3 miles to the Harris-Street Bridge, which will be on your right. Turn right just before the bridge to a parking area. The trail starts down by the Harpeth River beyond some vehicle-barrier boulders.

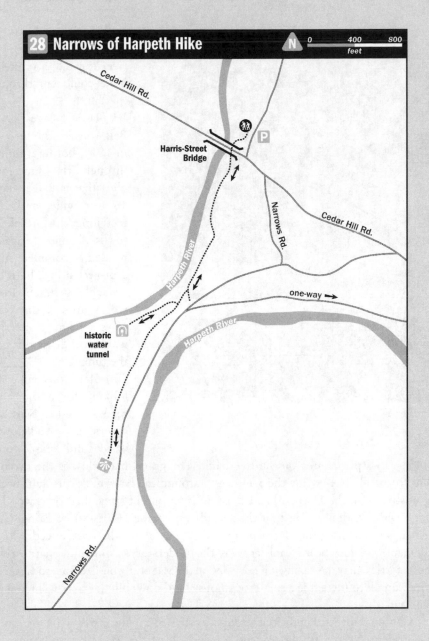

28 **Narrows of Harpeth Hike**

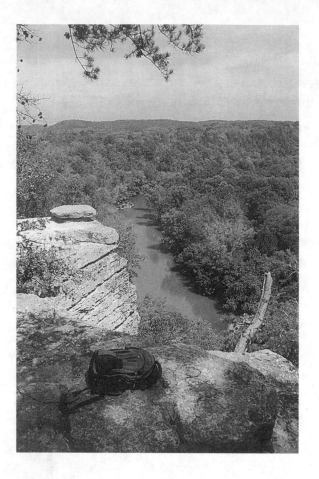

Vista of Harpeth River from atop the Narrows

his iron-ore industry by diverting water from the river through a tunnel—if he could cut through that bluff.

Using slave labor, Bell started the project in 1819, boring a tunnel through the limestone bluff that is 8 feet high, 16 feet wide, and 290 feet long. Just think of the skill and fortitude needed to complete such a project using the tools available then! The iron-works around the Narrows are long gone, but water still flows through the tunnel.

Start this hike by looking for a sign that reads, "Trail to Narrows at Bridge." Head downward and past some boulders to a picnic area on the riverbank. The gravel bar below is the takeout point for paddlers enjoying the 5-mile trip around the Narrows. Turn left, heading upstream on the Harpeth, and cross an intermittent streambed on a wooden bridge with handrails. The trail then heads under the Harris-Street Bridge and keeps upstream along the Harpeth, a good 50 feet above the river in cedar, oak, and maple woods; beard cane crowds the understory. Look out on the river where turtles may be lazing in the sun on logs. Soon you'll come to a rocky ravine: uphill to the left is a small rock house, and downhill the river is lined with small outcrops.

Continue forward and circle around a wooded ravine, crossing its low point on a bridge of cedar trunks. Ascend to walk along the base of a bluffline with many small rock houses. Shortly, you'll reach a gap and trail junction at 0.4 miles. To your left, one trail leads a short distance to the canoe put-in. Another trail heads to the Narrows overlook. And a third trail leads right, downhill on an old wagon road toward the tunnel. Turn right and descend on the old wagon road

into a flat where huge Eastern cottonwoods and sycamores tower over lush under-
brush. Soon you'll reach the pool created by the outflow from Montgomery Bell's
tunnel; this is a popular fishing hole. You can peer into the tunnel and appreciate
the hard work that was required to make it.

Backtrack 0.2 miles to the previous trail junction and take the trail uphill to
the overlook. Several wooden steps take you to the top of the bluff, then the walking is easy. Short side trails lead to the bluffline. Continue forward as the trail rises
among shortleaf pine and cedar to a clear overlook 0.3 miles from the junction.
Here, you can look down on the Harpeth River and the farm and hill country
through which it flows. You also can see both sides of the Harpeth and, to the
northeast, the white Harris-Street Bridge from where you came. On warm weekends, paddlers below drift down the river. The trail continues just a short distance
beyond the overlook to dead-end at private property. Backtrack 0.6 miles to the
trailhead.

NEARBY/RELATED ACTIVITIES

Here at the Narrows of Harpeth, you can make a 5-mile canoe trip without need-
ing a shuttle, using the trail described above. If you don't have a canoe, there are
several liveries in the area, such as Tip-A-Canoe, (800) 550-5810. For more information about the state historic area, visit **www.tnstateparks.com.**

29 NATHAN BEDFORD FORREST FIVE MILE LOOP

KEY AT-A-GLANCE INFORMATION

LENGTH: 4.9 miles

CONFIGURATION: Loop

DIFFICULTY: Moderate

SCENERY: Oak forests, shady hollows, big river

EXPOSURE: Mostly shady

TRAFFIC: Not much, some on nice weekends

TRAIL SURFACE: Leaves, moss, rocks, dirt

HIKING TIME: 2.7 hours

ACCESS: No fees or permits required

MAPS: Nathan Bedford Forrest Trail Map, available at visitor center

FACILITIES: Restrooms, water at visitor center

SPECIAL COMMENTS: This is just one loop among 20-plus miles of trails here.

IN BRIEF

This loop hike at Nathan Bedford Forrest State Park is an underused path at an underused state park. The terrain here will surprise you. Set among steep hills and deep hollows beside the wide Tennessee River, this trail is rich not only in natural beauty but in Tennessee history as well.

DESCRIPTION

Come to Nathan Bedford Forrest State Park if you're ready to embark on an adventurous mission from Nashville and learn a lot about the beauty and history of Tennessee. You have my guarantee as a native Tennessean that this 3,000-acre scenic swath will not disappoint you. For starters, it has 20 miles of well-marked, well-maintained, but little-trod trails. The trail system is situated on the western bank of the Tennessee River, which at this point is dammed as Kentucky Lake. Hardwood-covered hills rise 300 feet above the big river. Clear streams cut through surprisingly steep hollows.

Pilot Knob is the beginning point for the trail system. This high point is named for its use as a point of reference for riverboat pilots

GPS Trailhead Coordinates

UTM Zone (WGS84) 16S

Easting   0412270

Northing   3994020

Latitude   N 36° 5' 19.4"

Longitude   W 87° 58' 27.3"

Directions

From Exit 172 on I-40 west of Nashville, take TN 46 north 4.4 miles to US 70 Business west near Dickson. Stay on US 70 Business west 1.3 miles to US 70 west. Turn left and stay on US 70 west 40 miles to US 70 Business west into the town of Camden. From the town square at the Benton County Courthouse, take TN 191 north 8 miles to Nathan Bedford Forrest State Park. Stop at the park office and get a trail map. Continue forward beyond the park office to the Interpretive Center atop Pilot Knob. The trail starts on the left side of the building.

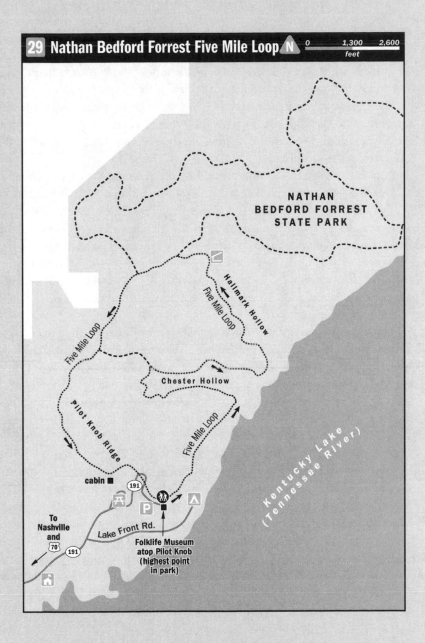

29 Nathan Bedford Forrest Five Mile Loop

N

0   1,300   2,600
feet

NATHAN
BEDFORD FORREST
STATE PARK

Hallmark Hollow

Five Mile Loop

Five Mile Loop

Chester Hollow

Five Mile Loop

Pilot Knob Ridge

Kentucky Lake
(Tennessee River)

cabin ■

191

Five Mile Loop

P

To
Nashville
and

70   191

Lake Front Rd.

Folklife Museum
atop Pilot Knob
(highest point
in park)

plying the Tennessee River below. I will admit this place is a little outside the 60-mile parameter of this book, but the trail system is too good to be overlooked.

Now, to the trails. A few of the shorter trails are isolated walks, and the rest are laid out in a series of interconnected loops. Loop hikes can range from 3 to 15 miles in length; backpackers use some of the longer loops for overnight camping. The following trail description is of the Five Mile Loop. Adventurous hikers, however, can look at the park map and come up with loops of varying lengths. During winter and early spring, hikers will be able to enjoy river views. In spring, visitors will see wildflowers in the hollows. In the summer, hikers will want to hit the trail early in the morning.

Before starting the hike, walk around to the river side of the building and gain far-reaching views of the Tennessee River and points east. Begin the Five Mile Loop, marked with orange metal blazes, atop Pilot Knob. Descend northeast atop a steep and surprisingly narrow ridgeline shaded by tall oaks. Notice that the trail bed is often lined with moss. Winter views of the river are off to your right. Drift downward, finally curving into Chester Hollow, originally called Cherry Hollow. This area was named for a fellow named Cherry, who lent his name to all sorts of area landmarks. Later, some errant map maker named it Chester Hollow—and the name stuck.

The path heads up the southern side of Chester Hollow, crossing over streambeds draining Pilot Knob Ridge. If the water is flowing, it will be surprisingly clear. Beech and tulip trees, along with omnipresent oaks, adorn the flat. Work up the hollow to make a trail junction at mile 1.5; signs indicate that the Five Mile Loop keeps to the right. Stay to your right and head east, out of Chester Hollow, where fingerlike flats extend into the hills. You'll arrive near the Tennessee River, only to turn away. Hikers could cut through some trees to reach the water's edge. The trail then curves into Hallmark Hollow, away from the river. Step over a few streambeds while working up the ever-narrowing hollow. Suddenly, the trail ascends a rib ridge to gain 200 feet in 0.1 mile. The rib ridge levels out to reach a backpacker's trail shelter at mile 2.8. Beyond this three-sided wooden structure, continue uphill at a more reasonable grade to soon arrive at a trail junction.

At the junction, the Five Mile Loop turns left. Begin following the main ridgeline of the park, which roughly parallels the north–south direction of the Tennessee River that you can see in winter from this ridge. The path undulates to reach another junction at mile 3.7. The Three Mile Loop joins here, also returning to Pilot Knob. Stay forward, though, and follow the orange blazes. The ridgetop trail begins curving southeast onto Pilot Knob Ridge, and other roads join the main path. Parts of the wide, roadlike trail have been cleared. Pass a park resident cabin on your right at mile 4.4, and descend from the cabin area to reach Pilot Knob Road. Pass around the metal gate, cross the road, and begin climbing toward Pilot Knob. Soon join Pilot Knob Road for the last ascent to the parking area and the end of the Five Mile Loop.

NEARBY/RELATED ACTIVITIES

Nathan Bedford Forrest State Park makes for a great overnight destination, offering camping, cabins, and outdoor activities. Anglers and boaters love the proximity of Kentucky Lake. The Nathan Bedford Forrest Interpretive Center, atop Pilot Knob, provides interesting information about the riverboat days on the Tennessee and the life of Confederate General Nathan Bedford Forrest, who fought one of the Civil War's most fascinating battles in this vicinity. Furthermore, this state park has two excellent campgrounds, including one situated directly on the banks of the Tennessee River. Having written seven campground guidebooks, I can say with authority that these sites are some of the finest in the Southeast.

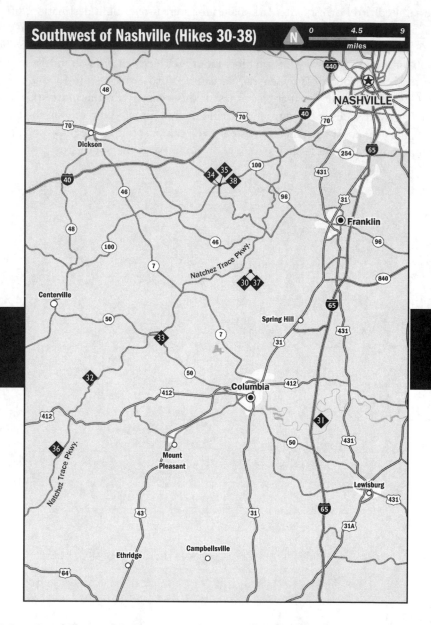

Southwest of Nashville (Hikes 30-38)

0   4.5   9
miles

N

NASHVILLE

440

48

70

70

70

Dickson

40

100

254

65

34 35
38

431

46

96

31

Franklin

48

100

46

96

7

Natchez Trace Pkwy.

840

30 37

Centerville

65

50

Spring Hill

431

33

7

31

32

50

Columbia

412

412

412

31

50

Natchez Trace Pkwy.

36

Mount
Pleasant

Lewisburg

65

431

43

31

31A

Ethridge

Campbellsville

64

30 Burns Branch There-and-Back 126
31 Cheeks Bend Bluff View Trail 129
32 Devils Backbone Loop 133
33 Gordon House and Ferry Site Walk 137
34 Horseshoe Trail 141

35 Lakes of Bowie Loop..................... 144
36 Meriwether Lewis Loop.................. 148
37 Old Trace–Garrison Creek Loop 152
38 Perimeter Trail 156

SOUTHWEST
INCLUDING COLUMBIA, FAIRVIEW, AND FRANKLIN

30 BURNS BRANCH THERE-AND-BACK

KEY AT-A-GLANCE INFORMATION

LENGTH: 2.8 miles
CONFIGURATION: There-and-back
DIFFICULTY: Easy
SCENERY: Wooded stream valley
EXPOSURE: Mostly shady
TRAFFIC: Quiet during the week, moderate on weekends
TRAIL SURFACE: Dirt, rocks
HIKING TIME: 1.3 hours
ACCESS: No fees or permits
MAPS: Natchez National Scenic Trail, Leipers Fork District
FACILITIES: Picnic tables at trailhead and trail-turnaround point; restrooms and water 2 miles north of trailhead on Natchez Trace Parkway at Garrison Creek

IN BRIEF

You will be surprised at this little gem of a hike in hilly country south of Nashville. Follow a portion of the Natchez Trace National Scenic Trail along a pretty creek up to a ridge that marks the Tennessee Valley Divide and the highest point along the entire Natchez Trace Parkway. Crystal-clear Burns Branch flows below gray-trunked beech trees shading the stream and much of the intimate valley through which the trail passes.

DESCRIPTION

This trail is mostly level or uphill. It gains 300 feet as it heads up the Burns Branch valley on its way to Duck River Ridge and the Tennessee Valley Divide. When you make it to the top, though, it is downhill all the way back. Duck River Ridge divides the watersheds of the Tennessee and Cumberland rivers: the waters north of the ridge, such as Burns Branch, flow into the Cumberland River, while the waters south of the ridge flow south into the Duck River and eventually the Tennessee River. Auto travelers will not notice the divide as readily as hikers will. This divide, which was very important to early northbound Trace travelers, marked the end of Chickasaw Indian

GPS Trailhead Coordinates

UTM Zone (WGS84) 16S
Easting   0495130
Northing   3967020
Latitude   N 35° 50' 57.2"
Longitude W 87° 3' 13.7"

Directions

From Exit 192 on Interstate 40 west of downtown Nashville, take McCrory Lane 4 miles south to intersect TN 100. Turn right and immediately pick up the Natchez Trace Parkway. Head south on the parkway 17 miles to the Burns Branch parking area on your left. The Natchez Trace National Scenic Trail heads in both directions. Take the scenic trail south, heading toward the Tennessee Valley Divide.

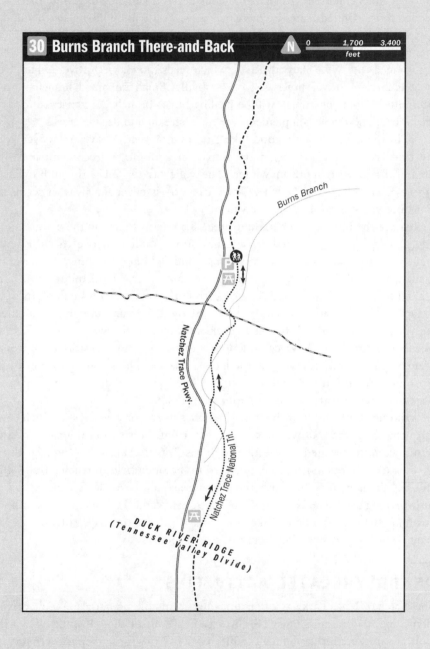

30 Burns Branch There-and-Back

N

0   1,700   3,400
feet

Burns Branch

Natchez Trace Pkwy.

Natchez Trace National Trl.

DUCK RIVER RIDGE
(Tennessee Valley Divide)

Territory and the relative nearness of Nashville. Later, in 1805, this territory south of the Tennessee River Divide, considered a vast howling wilderness, was deeded to the United States by the Chickasaw. You will be hiking southbound.

Naturally speaking, Burns Branch is one of Middle Tennessee's more scenic streams. Its clear waters, flowing over small rock ledges, feed Leipers Fork, which in turn feeds the West Harpeth River, which feeds the Harpeth River, which feeds the Cumberland River northwest of Nashville. Small unnamed branches, some intermittent, some perennial, will be feeding Burns Branch. An attractive forest of beech, oak, and maple complements the main stream and its side creeks.

This path makes for a good hike any time of year. Heavy tree cover keeps the trail cool in the summer and colorful in autumn. A freeze will make the stream glisten even more in winter. The valley is loaded with wildflowers in spring. Even though the Natchez Trace Parkway is never far away, it seems distant once you enter this attractive valley.

Leave the Burns Branch parking area, heading upstream in the margin alongside a field and the wooded streamside. Soon you'll pass over a clear feeder branch on a wooden bridge, entering a second field and reaching a quiet gravel road. Span Burns Branch on the road bridge and reenter woodland to cross Burns Branch on a footbridge. You'll squeeze through a wetland with small bluffs of the stream to your left and the parkway to your right. You are now in the middle of the valley, among smooth-trunked beech trees that shade swaying grasses. Crisscross the stream a few times and notice the small cascades formed by Burns Branch, sliding and dropping over ledge after ledge. The stream crossings can be dry-footed in all but the wettest of times. Keep an eye out, as the trail passes a large pool at the bottom of a four-foot waterfall.

Intermittent and flowing side branches form tiny valleys of their own, through which the trail winds. Climb away from the stream on a steep hillside, gaining a more elevated perspective of Burns Branch, before passing a small picnic area near an open field. Keep forward in the open field to reach a trail sign at mile 1.4. This high point marks the Tennessee Valley Divide. To the right is an auto-parking area. The Natchez Trace National Scenic Trail continues south, but this hike turns around here. Take your time on the return trip, noticing the intimate details of this small but beautiful streamshed.

NEARBY/RELATED ACTIVITIES

The Natchez Trace Parkway offers not only scenic hiking but also scenic driving, picnicking, and insights into U.S. history. Every bit of the 440 miles is worth a look. For more information, call (800) 305-7417 or visit **www.nps.gov/natr.**

CHEEKS BEND BLUFF VIEW TRAIL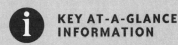

IN BRIEF

Explore this recent addition to the Tennessee State Natural Areas holdings, Cheeks Bend. Part of the 2,135-acre Duck River State Natural Area Complex, the trail travels along a bluff overlooking the Duck River and includes a special surprise—a side trip through a cave, where you can enter on a bluff top and emerge near the Duck at the base of the bluff.

DESCRIPTION

This trail leads to a cave with a 100-foot-or-so passage that leads from a river bluff overlooking the Duck River to the base of the same bluff. If you are afraid of the dark, bring a flashlight, though one is not necessary. The Cheeks Bend Vista Trail starts on the west side of the road. Begin following a singletrack path into the woods to reach a trailside kiosk showing the trail and giving information about the Duck River Complex. This complex is an agglomeration of six separate natural areas collectively within the Yanahli Wildlife Management Area. All are located in the Duck River Basin and include Columbia Glade, Sowell Mill, Rummage Cave, Howard Bridge

KEY AT-A-GLANCE INFORMATION

LENGTH: 1.8 miles
CONFIGURATION: Balloon
DIFFICULTY: Easy
SCENERY: River bluff, cedar woods, cave, riverside
EXPOSURE: Mostly shady
TRAFFIC: Not much
TRAIL SURFACE: Rocks, dirt
HIKING TIME: 1 hour
ACCESS: No fees or permits
MAPS: Available at www.tennessee .gov/environment/na/natareas/ duckriv/cheeksbend.pdf
FACILITIES: None

Directions

From Exit 46 on I-65, take TN 99, Sylvester Chunn Pike, east to US 431. Turn right, and take US 431 about 6 miles to reach Jordan Road. Turn right on Jordan Road (the left turn at this intersection is Wiles Lane). Follow Jordan Road west, crossing the Duck River (along the way, Jordan Road becomes Sowell Mill Pike). Watch for the left turn onto gravel Cheeks Bend Road 0.8 miles after crossing the Duck River on Sowell Mill Pike. Follow Cheeks Bend Road 0.9 miles to the trailhead.

GPS Trailhead Coordinates

UTM Zone (WGS84) 16S
Easting   0510440
Northing   3935820
Latitude   N 35° 34' 3.8"
Longitude   W 86° 53' 6.0"

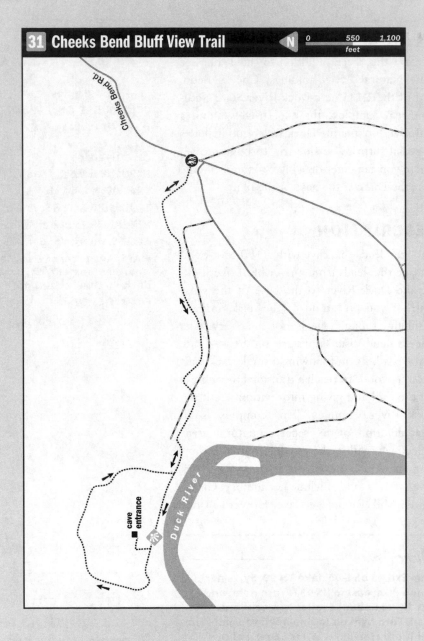

Glades, and Moore Lane, in addition to Cheeks Bend. This part of the Duck River is significant, as 13 of the 30 miles of the state scenic-river portion of the Duck are located here.

The blue-blazed track descends into oak–hickory–cedar woods, picking up an old roadbed. Here, the path makes an abrupt left turn, leaving the roadbed to cross a wet-weather branch. It then continues downhill, only to recross the branch just above a multitiered waterfall that likely won't fall at all in late summer and autumn. The Duck River will be visible through the trees in the winter.

Curve around to cross another wet-weather branch, and on your left you'll see the Duck River, which is a good 30 feet below the trail but can be accessed here. Just work your way down to reach some riverside rock outcrops that make for ideal sunning spots. Turtles know these are good sunning spots too; you'll see them splashing into the river as you head down. This isn't the ideal swimming hole, though, as the river is strongly sweeping around the bend here.

The path now ascends among pale rock outcrops as it works to the top of a bluff. Reach the loop portion of the trail at 0.6 miles. Continue forward, still stairstepping up the bluff, gaining obscured views of the river below. Ferns and mosses offer green contrast to the white outcrops, and cedars cling to shallow soils on the bluff. Reach the edge of the bluff, and you can look downriver to the southwest toward Interstate 65, which isn't visible but is audible.

The bluff levels off and reaches a junction. Watch carefully here for a cedar tree banded with both blue and red stripes. To reach the cave, turn right here and follow the red blazes away from the river and down to a cave entrance that's not visible from where you stand. The cave entrance is nearly square and big enough for a man to stand in. Follow the cave at a downhill angle, as the passage narrows and the world darkens. During summer, the temperature in the cave here can be 20 to 30 degrees cooler than it is outside. At this point, give your eyes time to adjust and you will be able to see, as light is coming from the passage that you just entered and also from the passage through which you will emerge—if you are tough enough to continue. As you continue downward, you will see other, smaller water-carved passages merging into the main cave. The cave opening down here is far taller than it is wide. You literally went under the bluff that you walked to get here. The Duck is still a good 30 feet or so below the lower cave opening. The track to the river from this point is rough and often muddy. However, you can explore in either direction along the base of the bluff. Backtrack up the cave and see how the upper entrance looks much different than the emergence of the lower entrance.

Return to the main trail and keep along the bluff, where you can see fields and woods across the river. At 0.8 miles, the trail turns away from the Duck, passing through a good spring-wildflower area before stairstepping over more outcrops to reach a high point. From there, work downhill while passing linear sinks. Complete the loop portion of the hike at 1.2 miles, then backtrack to the trailhead. Or maybe you'll make one more pass through the cave—like I did!

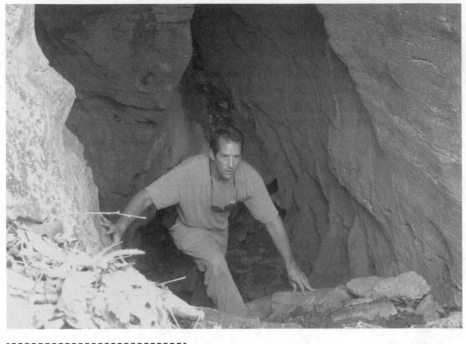

Author emerging from riverside cave

NEARBY/RELATED ACTIVITIES

Canoeing the Duck River lends a different perspective to this beautiful valley. River Rats canoe operation is located at the intersection of TN 99 and US 431, which you will pass on the way to Cheeks Bend. (There are two intersections of US 431 and TN 99; River Rats is at the more southerly one.) They offer canoe rentals and shuttles on the Duck. River Rats can be reached at (931) 381-2278 or **www.riverratcanoe.com.**

DEVILS BACKBONE LOOP 32

IN BRIEF

This hike traverses one of Tennessee's newer designated state natural areas. Conveniently located adjacent to the Natchez Trace Parkway, this preserve makes a loop through a seldom-traveled hardwood forest. The path stays in the center of the preserve, exuding an aura of wildness that makes even wintertime views of surrounding hills seem in the back of beyond.

DESCRIPTION

The name Devils Backbone conjures up an array of images in your mind—a hellish maze of rocks or maybe a menacing ridge of stone. But this name was actually inspired by the adjacent Natchez Trace. In the early 1800s, during the heyday of traveling the Trace from Natchez, Mississippi, to Nashville, an arduous trip was virtually assured. Flooded rivers, robbers, bad weather, hostile Native Americans, and the rigors of day-after-day, self-propelled travel made the journey challenging. The perils that befell Natchez Trace travelers were said to be the work of the devil, and the Devils Backbone sprang up as a nickname for the Trace.

Today, Devils Backbone seems as little used as the original Trace was after the advent of steamboats. The site, protected as a Tennessee State Natural Area in 1997 and dedicated

KEY AT-A-GLANCE INFORMATION

LENGTH: 2.7 miles
CONFIGURATION: Loop
DIFFICULTY: Easy to moderate
SCENERY: Hardwood forest, creek-filled hollow
EXPOSURE: Nearly all shady
TRAFFIC: You will likely have this trail to yourself
TRAIL SURFACE: Grass, moss, leaves, dirt
HIKING TIME: 1.3 hours
ACCESS: No fees or permits
MAPS: Parkway map available at www.nps.gov/natr
FACILITIES: Restrooms, water 15 miles north on Natchez Trace Parkway
SPECIAL COMMENTS: Consider traveling 2.2 miles south on Parkway to enjoy Fall Hollow Trail too.

Directions

From Exit 192 on I-40 west of downtown Nashville, take McCrory Lane 4 miles south to intersect TN 100. Turn right and immediately pick up the Natchez Trace Parkway. Head south on the parkway 48 miles to the signed right turn into Devils Backbone State Natural Area, on your right.

GPS Trailhead Coordinates

UTM Zone (WGS84) 16S
Easting 0465200
Northing 3942970
Latitude N 35° 34' 3.8"
Longitude W 87° 23' 2.1"

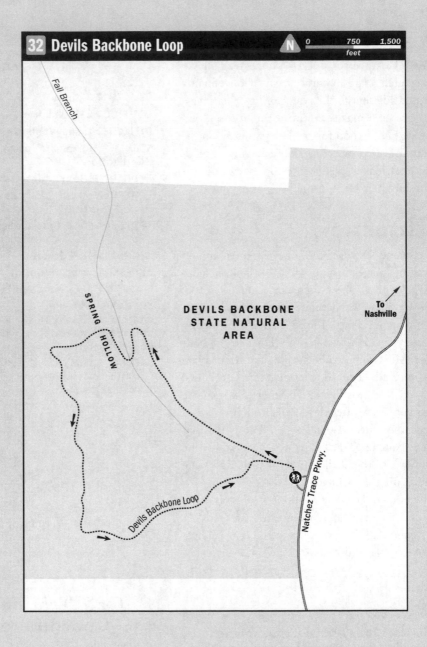

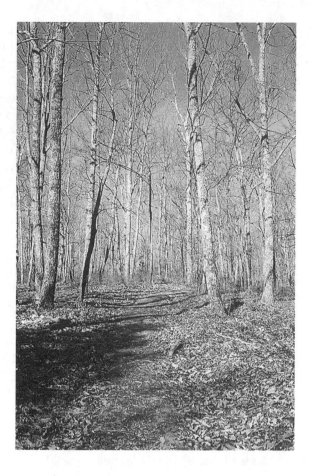

Lonely trail among winter hardwoods

in 2001, has an excellent loop trail through upland forest types of the Western Highland Rim. The Tennessee Natural Areas Program was established in 1971 by the state legislature, and since then 62 state natural areas have been established. The state of Tennessee doesn't own all the lands; rather it works with local, state, and federal agencies, as well as private landowners, in managing these sites. The goal is to attain adequate representation of all natural communities that comprise the landscape of the Volunteer State and provide long-term protection for rare, endangered, and threatened plant and animal life. Little exotic-plant invasion and good representation of tree species make the Devils Backbone a superior state natural area.

A hiker-registration book is at the trailside kiosk. Make sure to register—the more visitors this state-owned area gets, the greater the likelihood that it will remain preserved. Enter a lush hardwood forest comprised mostly of oaks on a singletrack path marked by white blazes. At 0.1 mile, the trail picks up an old woods road and turns left, slicing between steep and deep hollows. The trail bed of grass and moss indicates the infrequent use of this path, though the white blazes on trailside trees clearly mark the trail. It is easy to see why early Trace travelers stayed on the ridgelines, as trekking up and down the desiccated ravines would become tiresome.

At 0.4 miles, the loop portion of the trail begins. Stay to your right and work mostly downhill along another ridgeline. Notice that most of the trees here are chestnut oak, which is easily identified by its thick leaves with wavy edges. Chestnut oaks range from Maine to Mississippi, thriving in dry, rocky upland soils such as on this ridge. Since the demise of the American chestnut, the chestnut oak's density and distribution has increased. The nuts of the chestnut oak are favored by wildlife, and because of its high tannin content the tree's bark was once used for tanning leather.

The trail descends into Spring Hollow, reaching Fall Branch. Circle back to the left and step over Fall Branch at mile 1. The clarity of the stream allows you to peer into the water and look for underwater life. Ahead, cross a feeder branch on a footbridge, and head up the hollow to step over a third branch. The trail then curves back down Spring Hollow—this path is one of exploration, not expediency. This bottomland is rife with wildflowers in spring. Beech trees, which shade the hollow, love well-drained, moist soils like those in Spring Hollow. In fall, squirrels, raccoons, and other mammals gorge on beechnuts. As is often seen, the smooth trunks of beech trees prove irresistible for some folks who like to carve dates and names in them.

Climb out of Spring Hollow by switchbacks, returning to the oak-dominated ridgeline at mile 1.4. Turn left onto an old roadbed. (The seemingly endless forest and distant hills radiate a wildness that belies the size of the 950-acre natural area.) Undulate along the ridgeline, looking down into the hollows where small streamlets gather and feed Big Swan Creek to the west. The path curves back to the east, intersecting the beginning of the loop at 2.3 miles. From here, turn right and backtrack 0.4 miles to the trailhead.

NEARBY/RELATED ACTIVITIES

Just 2.1 miles south on the Natchez Trace is Fall Hollow Waterfall. A short paved trail leads to the top of this cascade.

GORDON HOUSE AND FERRY SITE WALK   33

IN BRIEF

This relatively short walk is laced with history. Located just off the Natchez Trace Parkway near Columbia on the banks of the Duck River, the trail first passes by the 200-year-old Gordon House. It then picks up a section of the Old Trace, following the actual route taken by Americans of long ago. The trail ends at the edge of the Duck River, where a ferry operated for nearly a century during the 1800s.

DESCRIPTION

The Natchez Trace follows an old path first used by buffalo and then by Native Americans who followed the animals. Later, as the United States began to be settled, farmers floated their crops down the waterways of the greater Mississippi River Valley to Natchez, Mississippi, or New Orleans to be sold. The strong currents that brought their flatboats down the river prevented their return float home, and the boats were dismantled and sold for lumber. The farmers then had a long walk up this Native American–buffalo path northward to their homes.

The United States realized the economic importance of the path and improved it to encourage trade. In 1800, the U.S. Army began establishing an official "Natchez Trace," pass-

KEY AT-A-GLANCE INFORMATION

LENGTH: 1 mile

CONFIGURATION: There-and-back

DIFFICULTY: Very easy

SCENERY: Fields, hardwood forest, creek, river

EXPOSURE: Mostly shady

TRAFFIC: Steady during good weather

TRAIL SURFACE: Asphalt, dirt

HIKING TIME: 30 minutes

ACCESS: No fees or permits

MAPS: Natchez Trace map available at www.nps.gov/natr

FACILITIES: Restrooms, covered picnic tables at parking area

Directions

From Exit 192 on I-40 west of downtown Nashville, take McCrory Lane 4 miles south to intersect TN 100. Turn right and immediately pick up the Natchez Trace Parkway. Head south on the parkway 34 miles to the Gordon House, on your left just past TN 50.

GPS Trailhead Coordinates

UTM Zone (WGS84) 16S

Easting   0476080

Northing 3952720

Latitude N 35° 43' 11.8"

Longitude W 87° 15' 51.7"

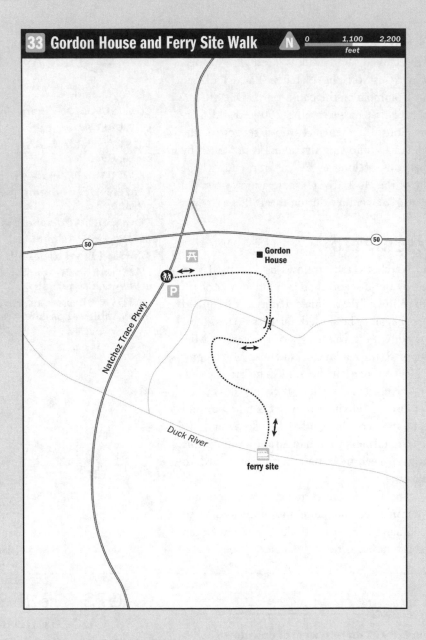

33 Gordon House and Ferry Site Walk

N

0   1,100   2,200
feet

50

50

Gordon
House

Natchez Trace Pkwy.

P

Duck River

ferry site

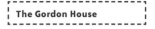
The Gordon House

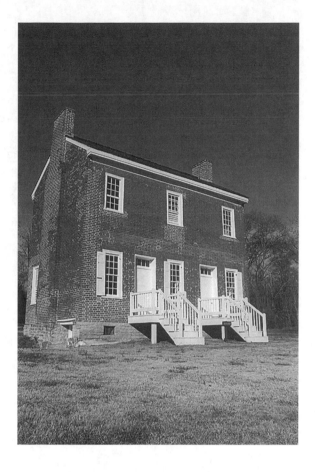

ing through Native American lands in Mississippi, Alabama, and Tennessee. Along the way, many inns, or stands as they were known, were established to feed and house travelers.

Around 1803, John Gordon, so-called Indian fighter and a friend of Andrew Jackson, obtained 600 acres along the Duck River in a land grant and began operating a ferry across the Duck near his homestead by the Old Trace. Before his ferry, travelers could cross the Duck only when it was low enough to be forded. In 1817, Gordon built himself and his wife a brick home, one of the first in the area. He died shortly after the home was built, but his wife continued to live there until her death in 1859. This is one of the few original buildings associated with the Old Trace.

Leave the parking area and follow the paved path to the Gordon House. The sturdy structure stands out on the landscape, no matter what the season, thanks in part to its white-paned windows that contrast with the red brick. John Gordon regularly saw the rise and fall of the Duck River through the seasons and smartly chose to build his home on this hill atop the floodplain.

The paved path ends at the house. Drop down the hill to your right, entering a grassy field where Gordon and his wife likely planted crops. Cross a bridge over Fattybread Creek. The name origin of this watercourse has been lost to time. An attractive grassy flat lies on the far side of the stream, and a contemplation bench overlooks the creek as it makes a bend toward the Duck River.

Pick up the Old Trace on the far side of Fattybread Branch. You can be sure that the soldiers who built this part of the road in 1802 drank from the branch. Think of all the travelers who, either coming or going, had the crossing of the

Duck River on their mind at this point. Follow the Old Trace as it passes over a hill and emerges onto another flat of grass broken by trees.

The trail skirts the edge of the flat and leads toward the Duck River. You'll reach a final level spot, which was the staging area for the ferry. Many a traveler, horseman, and farmer waited here. The dirt path continues down to the banks of the Duck. This usually clear, green, wide river is bordered in sycamore and hackberry.

Decades of off-and-on flooding have obliterated signs of the ferry operation, which ran from the early 1800s to 1896, when a bridge was built over the Duck. Gordon had to share his profits from the ferry with Chickasaw Chief George Colbert, who by treaty controlled ferries on Native lands. Now the Duck is easily crossed on the Natchez Trace Parkway and numerous other bridges. Life sure has changed over the past 200 years.

NEARBY/RELATED ACTIVITIES

The Natchez Trace Parkway offers other hiking trails, historical information, camping, and more. The Natchez Trace National Scenic Trail is just north of the Gordon House on TN 50. For more information about the parkway, visit **www .nps.gov/natr.**

HORSESHOE TRAIL 34

IN BRIEF

Horseshoe Trail is the forgotten path at Bowie Nature Park. The wide trail makes a loop in the southeast corner of the park. Though open to equestrians and hikers, the trail shows little signs of use by either group as it winds through a tall hardwood forest, crossing a small feeder branch of Little Turnbull Creek.

DESCRIPTION

Fairview resident Dr. Evangeline Bowie transformed the area that is this park from a barren, washed-out, abused land to the rich woodland we see today. With the help of her two sisters, "Van" Bowie reclaimed the land and planted trees to show how, given a chance, nature can restore itself to its former beauty.

Today, the park is not only a hiking destination but also a gathering place for Fairview's citizens to fish, picnic, and enjoy the sights and sounds of the great outdoors. The southeastern section of the park, through which the Horseshoe Trail travels, is reaping the benefits of the restoration and now stands tall in a forest of hardwoods such as oak and hickory. Small understory trees like dogwood, sourwood, and sassafras complement their tall brethren.

Sassafras trees are easy to identify, as their leaves have three basic shapes: oval, three-

KEY AT-A-GLANCE INFORMATION

LENGTH: 1.6 miles
CONFIGURATION: Loop
DIFFICULTY: Easy
SCENERY: Hardwood forest
EXPOSURE: Mostly shade
TRAFFIC: Solitude, nearly always
TRAIL SURFACE: Dirt, some loose rocks
HIKING TIME: 45 minutes
ACCESS: No fees or permits
MAPS: Bowie Nature Park Official Trail Map, available at trailhead and nature center
FACILITIES: Water spigot, restrooms, picnic area at trailhead
SPECIAL COMMENTS: Trail may close after rainy periods. Call (615) 799-5544, ext. 1, to confirm if trails are open.

Directions ⟶

From Exit 182 on I-40 west of downtown Nashville, take TN 96 south 5 miles to TN 100 at Fairview. Turn right on TN 100 and follow it 1.3 miles to Bowie Lake Road. Turn right on Bowie Lake Road and follow it 0.3 miles to the trailhead parking area on your right.

GPS Trailhead Coordinates

UTM Zone (WGS84) 16S
Easting 0476080
Northing 3980390
Latitude N 35° 58' 12.1"
Longitude W 87° 8' 8.3"

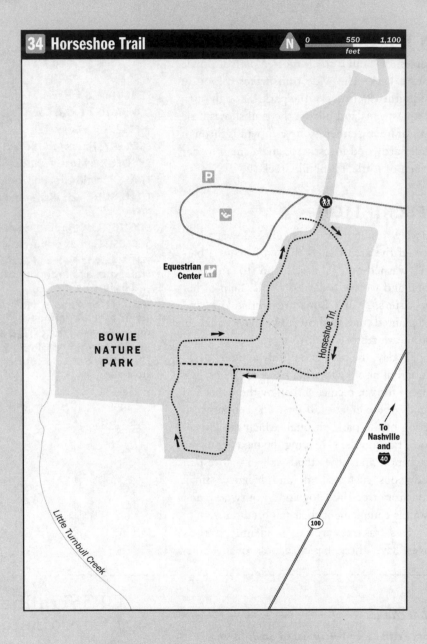

34 Horseshoe Trail

N

0　　550　　1,100
feet

P

Equestrian
Center

BOWIE
NATURE
PARK

Horseshoe Trl

To
Nashville
and
40

100

Little Turnbull Creek

lobed, and mitten-shaped. Mature sassafras trees have a reddish-brown, deeply furrowed bark. Sassafras are known for their aromatic scent: scratch the bark away from a twig, and the sweet smell is unmistakable. Native Americans used sassafras for medicinal purposes. Pioneers, and even people today, make tea by boiling sassafras roots, and birds eat the berries. The wood of sassafras shrinks when dried and is used for fence posts and hand tools.

The area dogwoods you see are Eastern flowering dogwoods. In spring, their white, creamy flowers brighten the woodlands where these trees grow. In summer, the green elliptical leaves with pale undersides give the dogwood away. In fall, it is identified by bright red berries (that are favored by birds) and scarlet leaves. And in winter, dogwoods can be identified by the rough brown bark that breaks into small square plates. Dogwoods grow from Ontario in the north to Florida in the south and extend eastward from the Atlantic Ocean all the way to central Texas. The wood of dogwood is very shock resistant and is used to make spools, pulleys, mallet heads, and jeweler's blocks. Native Americans used the bark and roots of dogwood to treat malaria and also extracted a red dye from dogwood roots.

Start the hike by leaving the trailhead parking area and walking 0.2 miles down Bowie Lake Road toward TN 100. Look right for the Horseshoe Trail sign and begin descending to reach a trail junction. This is the beginning of the loop portion of the Horseshoe Trail. Turn left and follow the orange blazes on the wide path, reaching the first intermittent stream branch at 0.4 miles. The streambed will likely be dry, except during rains. The Horseshoe Trail, like all other Bowie Nature Park trails, may be closed after heavy rains, so always call ahead before coming here.

Attractive hardwoods tower overhead as you continue. The path makes a sharp left where a more remote trail cuts the loop short. Stay left and parallel the park border, nearing pastureland; its openness contrasts greatly with the shady forest. Circle back down a north-facing slope rich with ferns to again reach the intermittent stream. Ascend into the only broken woods of the hike before reaching the beginning of the loop. Keep forward and reach Bowie Lake Road at 1.4 miles. Turn left and backtrack down the road to the trailhead parking area.

NEARBY/RELATED ACTIVITIES

This is more than a park with trails. Bowie Nature Park also has a nature center, several small lakes open to fishing, an elaborate playground for kids, and several picnic shelters. Consider making a day of it, and cook out. For more park information, visit **www.fairview-tn.org/bowiepark/index.html.**

35 LAKES OF BOWIE LOOP

KEY AT-A-GLANCE INFORMATION

LENGTH: 2.2 miles

CONFIGURATION: Loop

DIFFICULTY: Easy

SCENERY: Small lakes, pine woods

EXPOSURE: Part sun, part shade

TRAFFIC: Plenty of solitude during the week, some company on weekends

TRAIL SURFACE: Wood chips, pine needles, dirt

HIKING TIME: 1.2 hours

ACCESS: No fees or permits

MAPS: Bowie Nature Park Official Trail Map, available at trailhead and nature center

FACILITIES: Water spigot, restrooms, picnic area at trailhead

SPECIAL COMMENTS: Trail may close after rainy periods. Call (615) 799-5544, ext. 1, to confirm if trails are open.

IN BRIEF

This loop hike encompasses several short scenic trails of Bowie Nature Park, touring four of the preserve's lakes. The trails have good footing, are mostly level and wide, and are suitable for a family hike, especially for younger children. Wildlife can be abundant as well, with waterfowl in the lakes and deer and more in adjacent woods.

DESCRIPTION

This is a water- and wildlife-lover's walk that meanders by small lakes, beneath tall pines, and through quiet hollows. Take the Lake Van Trail, circling this attractive impoundment, and pick up the Loblolly Loop, passing by Upper Lake. Cross a spring branch to get to Lake Byrd and a picnic shelter. Circle by Lake Anna before returning to the trailhead, passing by Sycamore Springs, a chilly water source from the days when Bowie Nature Park was a farmstead.

Waterfowl enjoy the lakes, which also harbor fish and are open to fishing. Watch for land critters too. I have seen deer on nearly every visit here. Keep your eyes open as you walk along the edges of the lakes and edges where field and forest meet.

A number of trails wind through Bowie Nature Park; those in the heart of the park are

GPS Trailhead Coordinates

UTM Zone (WGS84)   16S

Easting   0487490

Northing   3980500

Latitude   N 35° 58' 14.2"

Longitude   W 87° 8' 18.8"

Directions

From Exit 182 on I-40 west of downtown Nashville, take TN 96 south 5 miles to TN 100 at Fairview. Turn right on TN 100 and follow it 1.3 miles to Bowie Lake Road. Turn right on Bowie Lake Road and follow it 0.3 miles to the trailhead parking area on your right.

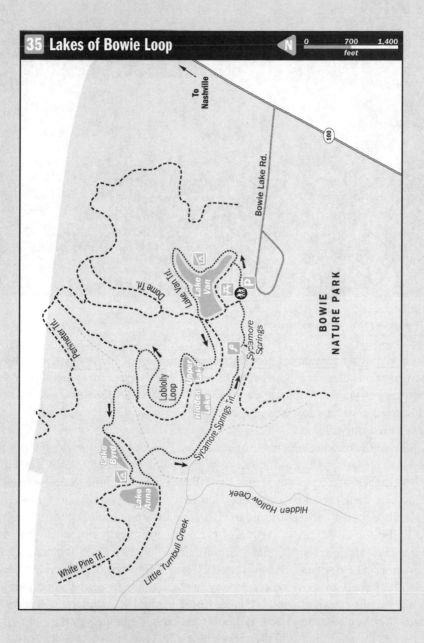

35 Lakes of Bowie Loop

N

0   700   1,400
feet

To Nashville

100

Bowie Lake Rd.

BOWIE NATURE PARK

Dome Trl.

Lake Van Trl.

Lake Van

Perimeter Trl.

Sycamore Springs

Loblolly Loop

Upper Lake

Hidden Lake

Sycamore Springs Trl.

Lake Byrd

Lake Anna

Hidden Hollow Creek

Little Turnbull Creek

White Pine Trl.

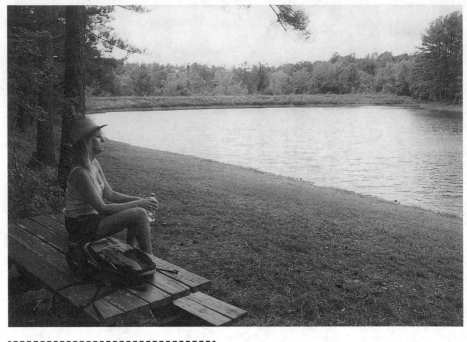

Overlooking Lake Anna on a summer day

designated as scenic trails. This hike traces a portion of the scenic trails, though you may want to create your own loop. In fact, there are so many small trails, you may make up your own loop just trying to follow this one. Don't worry, though— it's hard to get really lost here, especially if you have a park map, which can be picked up at the trailhead.

From the parking area near the restrooms, walk around a wooden fence past the small playground toward the Lake Van Trail. A signed path leads downhill a short distance to access the actual Lake Van Trail. Take the wide path to the right, with the clear lake to your left, and cross over a wooden bridge. Relaxed anglers are sometimes seen sitting in chairs beside a pole, waiting for a bream to tug under the cork. Pass a couple of picnic shelters and curve around a small embayment of the lake. A wetland community has grown up in the margins that are neither lake nor land, and birdhouses have been nailed into lakeside trees.

The Lake Van Trail makes its way along the length of the impoundment. Notice cattails growing along the lake. Come to the lake dam and continue forward. Now you're on the Loblolly Loop (the Dome Trail goes to the right). True to the trail's name, tall loblolly trees along this path tower overhead, swaying with any gust of wind. Curve around on an old woods road and soon reach Upper Lake, which is visible through the trees to your left.

Circle Upper Lake and stay in pine woods. Don't be surprised to hear a woodpecker here. The dry ravine to your left is an old, failed dam. An unsigned side trail soon leaves right. Stay with the main old-woods road and descend to another junction. Turn right here, looking for the sign that reads "To Twin Lakes." Descend to step over an intermittent streambed, then enter a small clearing on your right. This is deer country.

Before you know it, another lake appears—Lake Byrd. Walk across the dam of this lake and come to a picnic shelter at mile 1.4. This shelter overlooks the lake and makes a great midway picnic spot. Lake Anna is just a few steps down the trail beyond the picnic shelter. Here, the White Pine Trail leaves to the right. Stay left, though, and walk along the shore of Lake Anna for 75 yards. Here, take an acute left away from the lake, not crossing the earthen dam. Continue forward, and soon look for the sign indicating Sycamore Springs. Turn right toward Sycamore Springs and descend into a moisture-loving hardwood forest that contrasts greatly with the piney woods encountered earlier. The tree canopy soon opens in a storm-damaged section before reaching the easily identifiable Sycamore Springs. This clear water source had been bricked and concreted in days gone by. Look for frogs in the water. Stick your hand in it—you'll find that the water is quite chilly. Come to another junction just past the spring. The Three Sisters–Perimeter Trail leaves right. Stay left, ascending a hill to reach the trailhead, and complete the loop.

NEARBY/RELATED ACTIVITIES

This is more than a park with trails. Bowie Nature Park also has a nature center, several small lakes open to fishing, an elaborate playground for kids, and several picnic shelters. Consider making a day of it, and cook out. For more park information, visit **www.fairview-tn.org/bowiepark/index.html.**

36   MERIWETHER LEWIS LOOP

KEY AT-A-GLANCE INFORMATION

LENGTH: 3.5 miles

CONFIGURATION: Loop

DIFFICULTY: Easy to moderate

SCENERY: Ridge and streamside forest

EXPOSURE: Mostly shady

TRAFFIC: Moderate

TRAIL SURFACE: Dirt, rocks, leaves

HIKING TIME: 2 hours

ACCESS: No fees or permits

MAPS: Meriwether Lewis Site Hiking Trails, available at trailhead

FACILITIES: Restrooms, water at Meriwether Lewis campground during warm season, restrooms only in winter

SPECIAL COMMENTS: This loop is only one among several possible loop combinations at the Meriwether Lewis Monument site.

IN BRIEF

This hike is centered on Meriwether Lewis Monument, just off the Natchez Trace Parkway. Meriwether Lewis died here in 1809, during his return trip to Washington from St. Louis. The hike begins at Grinders Stand, follows the historic Trace for a mile down to attractive Little Swan Creek, and eventually loops back to the monument area.

DESCRIPTION

This loop hike travels some very historic ground. It was at Grinders Stand on the Natchez Trace, on October 11, 1809, where Meriwether Lewis died under circumstances that remain mysterious to this day. Following his famed expedition to the Pacific accompanied by William Clark, Lewis was appointed governor of Louisiana, which covered roughly 15 million acres, essentially the extent of the Louisiana Purchase. The government did not honor some of his expenses for the expedition, so Lewis decided to return to Washington to dispute them. He traveled south by water from St. Louis to the site of present-day Memphis, then headed east by land to avoid the British presence offshore, where he feared his expedition papers might be confiscated. Thus, he and a few companions found themselves on the

GPS Trailhead Coordinates

UTM Zone (WGS84) 16S

Easting 0458190

Northing 3929680

Latitude N 35° 30' 41.6"

Longitude W 87° 27' 40.0"

Directions ——————————→

From Exit 46 on I-65 south of downtown Nashville, take US 412 west 34 miles to the Natchez Trace Parkway, passing through Columbia. Turn right onto the parkway access road, then stay forward, heading to "Historical Exhibit" at Meriwether Lewis Monument. Park at area near log cabin on left.

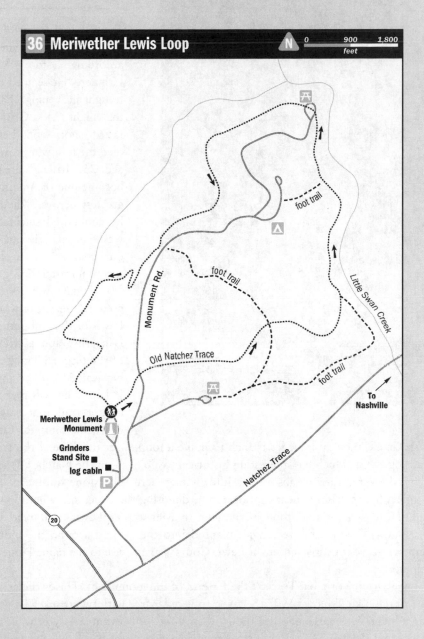

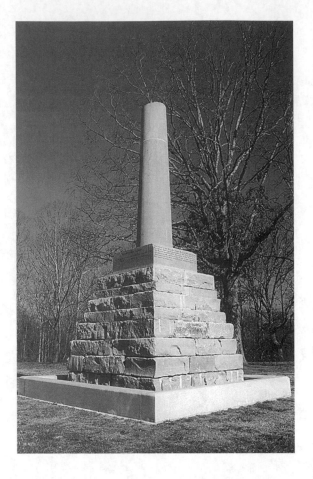

Meriwether Lewis
Monument

Trace. Lewis arrived first at Grinders Stand, where, according to Mrs. Grinder, "He seemed distraught all evening." Later that night, Mrs. Grinder heard shots and Lewis died the following day, at age 35, having already become one of America's greatest heroes. Whether he committed suicide or was murdered is one of our country's great historical uncertainties.

Today, visitors can go to the very spot where Lewis died. A monument is nearby, and a stretch of the original Trace can be walked for a mile. Hikers then will pick up a foot trail that travels down the bluffs of Little Swan Creek, then up a feeder branch to make a loop. Start this hike at the trailhead log cabin, which has interesting historical exhibits about the Natchez Trace.

Take some time to absorb the information here. The stone outline of the Grinders Stand cabin is near the log cabin, denoting the exact site where Lewis died. Head toward the stone monument to Meriwether Lewis, and read the inscriptions. The marble rectangles planted into the ground around the monument are graves of early settlers of Lewis County, giving rise to the name Pioneers Cemetery.

Pick up the original Trace at the far end of the monument. This is the actual start of the hike. Follow the Trace past a split cedar tree with two trunks. To your left, a hiker sign marks another trail; this is your return route. As you walk the Trace, consider how American history might have changed had Lewis walked the path you are on now, instead of having his journey cut short at Grinders Stand. Considering his fame and popularity after his Corps of Discovery mission to the Pacific, he might have become President. The Meriwether Lewis Monument, a shaft extending skyward, is broken off at the top, symbolizing a life of potential greatness cut short for reasons unknown.

The original Trace soon crosses Monument Road, then passes another trail leading left, a loop shortcut. The original Trace becomes gullied as it descends to Peavyhouse Hollow and Little Swan Creek, where it meets a foot trail at mile 1. Turn left onto the foot trail, and Little Swan Creek will be off to your right. Head downstream, soon climbing, as this side of the creek becomes a steep bluff. Reach a side trail leading left to the area campground. Keep forward in the Little Swan Creek valley, where views extend from the bluff. Soon you'll reach the picnic area. Walk across the picnic parking area, passing a copse of cedar trees at mile 1.7.

You'll enter the woods at a hiker trail sign with a couple of picnic tables off to your right. Now you're heading upstream along a noisy feeder branch of Little Swan Creek. The singletrack path works up the feeder-stream valley, circling into and out of side hollows. Turn away from the stream valley onto a hardwood ridge-line, reaching Monument Road at mile 2.7. Immediately turn away from the road, passing beneath a picnic table and overlook. Descend back into the feeder branch hollow by switchbacks and resume heading upstream in a fern-dotted flat, crossing the streambed twice in succession. Here, the streambed is normally dry. Switch-back out of the creekbed to emerge onto the original Trace near the Meriwether Lewis Monument at mile 3.5, ending the hike.

NEARBY/RELATED ACTIVITIES

The Meriwether Lewis Monument area has more than just hiking trails. The monument-area roads and nearby Natchez Trace are good for bicycling. And there's a quiet, first-rate campground here. Nearby is the Buffalo River, which is great for canoeing. Outfitters are located in nearby Hohenwald. Visit **www.nps .gov/natr** for more information.

37 OLD TRACE-GARRISON CREEK LOOP

KEY AT-A-GLANCE INFORMATION

LENGTH: 6.3 miles

CONFIGURATION: Balloon

DIFFICULTY: Moderate

SCENERY: Ridgetop and creekside forests

EXPOSURE: Mostly shady

TRAFFIC: Moderately busy on weekends

TRAIL SURFACE: Dirt, rocks

HIKING TIME: 3.5 hours

ACCESS: No fees or permits

MAPS: Natchez National Scenic Trail, Leipers Fork District

FACILITIES: Picnic tables at trailhead; restrooms, water at Garrison Creek, halfway through hike

SPECIAL COMMENTS: Trail passes through tunnel beneath parkway

IN BRIEF

Walk through time on this trek, picking up the original Natchez Trace, where travelers made their way from Natchez, Mississippi, to Nashville two centuries ago.

DESCRIPTION

The hike travels through varied environments on its journey from Burns Branch to Garrison Creek. The hike begins in quiet field and forest country on the Natchez Trace National Scenic Trail. The path heads up and down, winding in and out of small wooded coves, only to emerge onto the original Natchez Trace. It then makes a pleasant forest cruise on the longest section of Old Trace left in Tennessee, before taking a side path to a scenic overlook, where you can see the Garrison Creek valley and Middle Tennessee countryside.

Descend to Garrison Creek, picking up the Garrison Creek Loop Trail. Cross the clear stream twice before heading back toward the Old Trace. Here, the path takes an unexpected route, passing under the Natchez Trace Parkway via a modern tunnel built just for the hikers and equestrians who use this path. Climb a piney hillside before once again meeting the Old Trace, backtracking to the trailhead.

GPS Trailhead Coordinates

UTM Zone (WGS84) 16S

Easting   0496170

Northing 3968710

Latitude   N 35° 51' 52.8"

Longitude   W 87° 2' 31.6"

Directions

From Exit 192 on I-40 west of downtown Nashville, take McCrory Lane 5 miles south to intersect TN 100. Turn right and immediately pick up the Natchez Trace Parkway. Head south on the parkway 17 miles to the Burns Branch parking area on your left. The Natchez Trace National Scenic Trail heads in both directions. Take the scenic trail north, heading toward Garrison Creek.

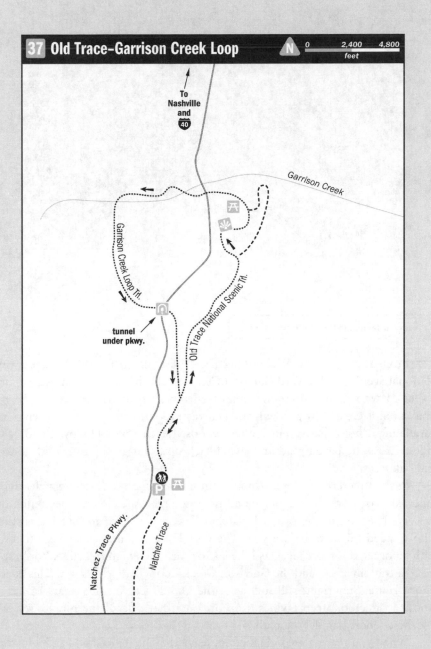

37 Old Trace–Garrison Creek Loop

N

0   2,400   4,800
feet

To
Nashville
and
40

Garrison Creek

Garrison Creek Loop Tr.

Old Trace National Scenic Tr.

tunnel
under pkwy.

Natchez Trace Pkwy.

Natchez Trace

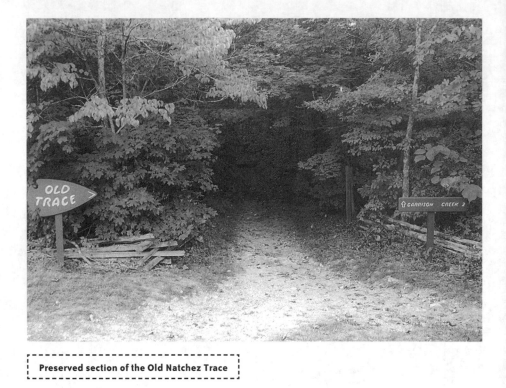

Preserved section of the Old Natchez Trace

From the Burns Branch parking area, head north on the Natchez Trace National Scenic Trail toward Garrison Creek. Walk the margin of a field to enter a slice of woodland and cross a small feeder branch of Burns Branch, where a small pool is created by a flow from a culvert; look for fish in here. Keep north, paralleling a horse pasture in broken woods. Reach Davis Hollow Road at 0.6 miles. Cross the paved road and switchback up a hill grown over with hickory and oak trees.

Begin a pattern of dipping in and out of coves before reaching a clearing at mile 1.3. To your left is a picnic and parking area. Ahead is the beginning of a preserved section of the original Natchez Trace. It is hard to imagine all those who treaded this path before you. The Old Trace is much wider here than the path before and is more level, as it keeps forward on a high ridgeline. You'll soon reach a trail junction, and the Garrison Creek Loop Trail leaves left. This is your return route. Stay right, still following the Old Trace, keeping near the heavily wooded ridgetop. Steep ravines drop off on either side of the now-rocky trail. Old wire fences parallel the path.

When you reach a second junction, leave the Old Trace and head left to the Garrison Creek Overlook. From here, you can see the valley to which you are headed. Make your way down to reach the Garrison Creek parking area at 3 miles. Here you'll find restrooms, a water spigot, and picnic tables. The main trail comes in from the right, just before reaching the building at the parking area.

The trail seems to die out in the grassy fields. Fear not and keep downhill, reaching Garrison Creek and some streamside picnic tables. Now, keep upstream along the edge of the field beside the creek, contemplating a garrison of soldiers who camped along this stream as they built the Old Trace 200 years ago. Pass under the bridge of the parkway and watch for a dirt path, leaving right, to cross Garrison Creek. This is the continuation of the Garrison Creek Loop Trail. This is a wet crossing, meaning you ain't gettin' across unless you get your feet wet. Consider taking off your shoes and barefooting it across the 15 feet of normally mid-shin-high water. As you ford, the clarity of the stream will surprise you. Back in their time, the soldiers who built the trail drank this water without purification or compunction. Those days are gone.

Keep upstream, in a sliver of woods between the creek and a field to your right. Enjoy an attractive and pleasant stroll before fording Garrison Creek at mile 3.8. Make a short but steep climb beyond the ford to reach the tunnel burrowing beneath the parkway. This short but exciting tunnel has an elevated sidewalk for pedestrians and a larger, lower, and wider way for horses. The trail then slabs the side of a ridgeline through piney woods, which gives way to hardwoods before reaching the Old Trace at mile 4.8. Turn right here, following the Old Trace 0.2 miles. Keep backtracking north on the Natchez Trace National Scenic Trail to reach the Burns Branch parking area at mile 6.3.

NEARBY/RELATED ACTIVITIES

The Natchez Trace Parkway offers not only scenic hiking, but also scenic driving, picnicking, and insights into American history. Visit **www.nps.gov/natr**.

38   PERIMETER TRAIL

 KEY AT-A-GLANCE INFORMATION

LENGTH: 5.1 miles

CONFIGURATION: Loop

DIFFICULTY: Moderate

SCENERY: Woodlands, small streamsheds

EXPOSURE: Part sun, part shade

TRAFFIC: Alone during the week, some trail users on weekends

TRAIL SURFACE: Dirt

HIKING TIME: 2.5 hours

ACCESS: No fees or permits

MAPS: Bowie Nature Park Official Trail Map available at trailhead and nature center

FACILITIES: Water spigot, restrooms, picnic area

SPECIAL COMMENTS: Trail may close after rainy periods. Call (615) 799-5544, ext. 1, to confirm if trails are open.

IN BRIEF

Operated by the town of Fairview, Bowie Nature Park traverses mildly rolling Middle Tennessee forestland not usually slated for preservation. The Bowie Sisters, longtime Fairview residents, rehabilitated this cut-over, burned-over, and eroded land, then deeded it to the town of Fairview. What remains today is an attractive forest with trees of differing ages, cut by clear creeks forming small valleys. The distance is the most challenging aspect of the hike.

DESCRIPTION

Parks historically have been created and preserved in large part due to the exceptional beauty of the land's physical features. In regard to beauty, Bowie Nature Park is in a league of its own. Land like Bowie Nature Park is typically used for farmland, pastureland, or is otherwise developed. In the past, this land was agriculturally mismanaged. But thanks to Evangeline Bowie and her two sisters, it was rehabilitated and deeded to the city of Fairview, which now runs the property as a park.

The Perimeter Trail, which makes a loop along the edge of the 800-acre park, is great for hikers wanting to extend their trips but not wanting to get on something too tough.

GPS Trailhead Coordinates

UTM Zone (WGS84) 16S

Easting 0487490

Northing 3980500

Latitude N 35° 58' 14.2"

Longitude W 87° 8' 18.8"

Directions ————————————➤

From downtown Nashville, head west on I-40 to Exit 182 and TN 96. Head south on TN 96 and drive 5 miles to TN 100 at Fairview. Turn right on TN 100 and follow it 1.3 miles to Bowie Lake Road. Turn right on Bowie Lake Road and follow it 0.3 miles to the trailhead parking area on your right.

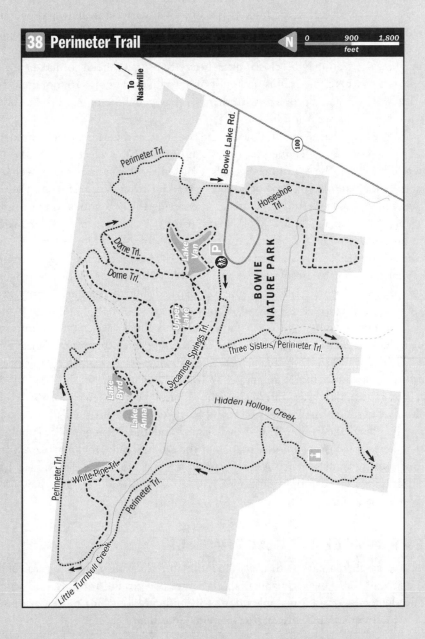

38 Perimeter Trail

N

0   900   1,800
feet

To Nashville

Perimeter Trl.

Bowie Lake Rd.

100

Horseshoe Trl.

Dome Trl.

Lake Van

P

Dome Trl.

BOWIE NATURE PARK

Upper Lake

Sycamore Springs Trl.

Three Sisters/Perimeter Trl.

Lake Byrd

Hidden Hollow Creek

Lake Anna

Perimeter Trl.

White Pine Trl.

Perimeter Trl.

Little Turnbull Creek

Though you may not always get a feel of being in the wild, the fields and woods of the park provide an ideal habitat for wildlife. The trail is a mixture of old woods roads and singletrack trail. Quiet hikers in early mornings and evenings are likely to spot deer that roam the park. Since much of the path is not canopied, I recommend hiking here during fall, winter, and spring—summer can be hot. Be aware that the trail may be closed after heavy rains; call ahead to make sure it's open. As a footnote, the trail is open not only to hikers but also to mountain bikers. I have never had a problem with them as they pedal the path, but you should listen for them on weekend hikes.

To start the Perimeter Trail, leave the trailhead and parking area behind and head west toward the Tennessee Valley Authority (TVA) electric line, keeping downhill to reach the Sycamore Springs Trail on the far side of the power line. Descend along an old road to soon reach a trail junction. Veer left onto the red-blazed Three Sisters–Perimeter Trail, soon entering thicker woods to reach Little Turnbull Creek at 0.5 miles. Work away from the creek in mixed hardwoods with many dogwoods, and again come to the TVA line. Veer left and cruise along the line 0.3 miles before reentering pine and oak woods with a broken canopy. The trail turns northwest and passes near Hidden Hollow Creek before reaching an old cemetery at mile 2.1. One grave is marked, but the rest are simply fieldstones languishing under the shade of dogwood trees.

Continue downhill and reach Little Turnbull Creek, a clear, rock-bottomed stream that's backed by stone bluffs. The creek can be dry-footed most times of the year. A foot trail heads upstream from the crossing. The Perimeter Trail briefly keeps downstream before climbing away from the watercourse and heading due east along the park border, intersecting the White Pine Trail. Keep forward as the trail moves through small valleys of mixed hardwoods and piney hills.

At mile 4, the Dome Trail leaves right, and the Perimeter Trail makes a U-turn left, soon passing another branch of the Dome Trail. Stay in broken woods before passing under the TVA line. Continue south to emerge at Bowie Lake Road at mile 4.9. Turn right on Bowie Lake Road and walk through the park to complete the loop.

NEARBY/RELATED ACTIVITIES

This is more than a park with trails. Bowie Nature Park also has a nature center, several small lakes open to fishing, an elaborate playground for kids, and several picnic shelters. Consider making a day of it, and cook out. For more park information, visit **www.fairview-tn.org/bowiepark/index.html**.

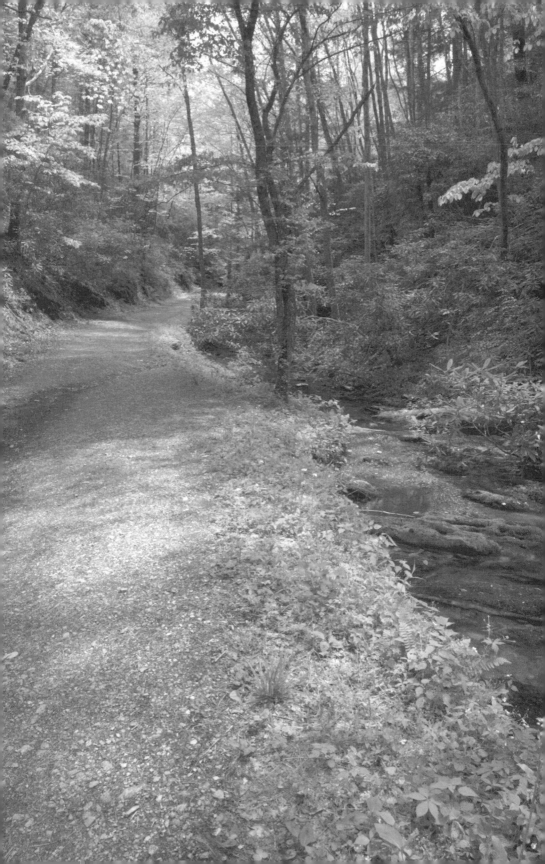

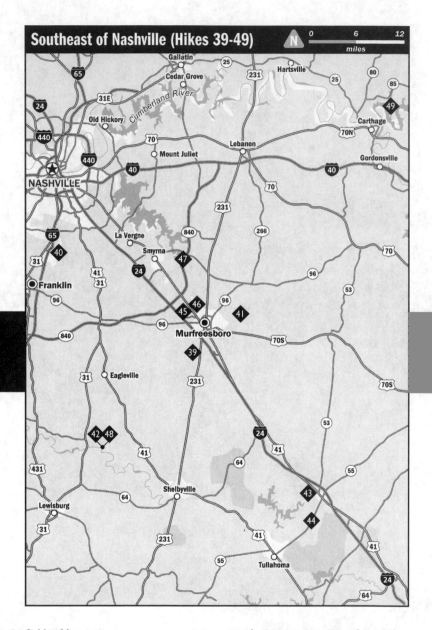

Southeast of Nashville (Hikes 39-49)

N   0   6   12
         miles

- Gallatin
- 25
- Hartsville
- 65
- 231
- Cedar Grove
- 25
- 80
- 85
- 31E
- Cumberland River
- 24
- Old Hickory
- 49
- 440
- 70
- Lebanon
- 70N
- Carthage
- 440
- Mount Juliet
- Gordonsville
- 40
- 40
- NASHVILLE
- 70
- 231
- 65
- La Vergne
- 840
- 266
- 70
- 40
- Smyrna
- 47
- 31
- 41
- 24
- 96
- 31
- 53
- Franklin
- 96
- 46
- 96
- 45
- 41
- 96
- 840
- Murfreesboro
- 70S
- 39
- 31
- Eagleville
- 231
- 70S
- 53
- 24
- 42
- 48
- 41
- 41
- 431
- 64
- 55
- Shelbyville
- 43
- Lewisburg
- 64
- 44
- 31
- 231
- 41
- 41
- 55
- Tullahoma
- 24
- 64

39 Barfield Wilderness Loop................ 162
40 Brenthaven Bikeway Connector.......... 166
41 Flat Rock Cedar Glades and Barrens Hike. 170
42 Old Mill Trail............................ 174
43 Old Stone Fort Loop 178
44 Short Springs State Natural Area Hike 182
45 Stones River Battlefield Loop 186
46 Stones River Greenway of Murfreesboro.. 190
47 Twin Forks Trail......................... 193
48 Wild Turkey Trail........................ 197

SOUTHEAST
INCLUDING BRENTWOOD, MURFREESBORO, AND SMYRNA

39 BARFIELD WILDERNESS LOOP

KEY AT-A-GLANCE INFORMATION

LENGTH: 2.5 miles

CONFIGURATION: Loop

DIFFICULTY: Easy to moderate

SCENERY: Hardwood and cedar forest

EXPOSURE: Mostly shady

TRAFFIC: Busy on weekends

TRAIL SURFACE: Asphalt, dirt, rocks

HIKING TIME: 1.3 hours

ACCESS: No fees or permits

MAPS: Available at Wilderness Station at trailhead

FACILITIES: Restrooms, water at Wilderness Station

SPECIAL COMMENTS: Backcountry camping is also allowed on this trail.

IN BRIEF

This hike loops through the naturally preserved portion of Barfield Crescent Park. It heads away from the Wilderness Station, an environmental education–activity center, and reaches the West Fork Stones River. From there, it skirts along the shore and bluff of this quintessential Middle Tennessee stream. The path then heads up to Marshall Knob and a stone fence, whose origin is the subject of debate.

DESCRIPTION

The city of Murfreesboro recognized the growing desire among its citizens for hiking trails. By expanding Barfield Crescent Park, the city's parks and recreation department added a 275-acre backcountry area, much of which borders the West Fork Stones River. The park's name comes from a Revolutionary War soldier, Frederick Barfield, who was given a land grant of nearly 3,000 acres on the West Fork Stones River. The West Fork is a changing stream—it can run nearly dry in late summer and be a torrent in winter. Nevertheless, the river remains a scenic centerpiece of the area.

This loop hike changes character frequently as well. It starts out as a paved path

GPS Trailhead Coordinates

UTM Zone (WGS84) 16S

Easting 0552790

Northing 3959300

Latitude N 35° 46' 41.6"

Longitude W 86° 24' 59.8"

Directions

From Exit 81A on Interstate 24 southeast of downtown Nashville, take US 231 south 1.7 miles to Barfield Crescent Road. Turn right on Barfield Crescent Road and follow it 0.8 miles to Barfield Crescent Park. Turn left into the park, then turn right after 0.3 miles and follow the signs to shortly reach the Wilderness Station. The loop starts in the upper left corner of the parking area as you look out from the Wilderness Station.

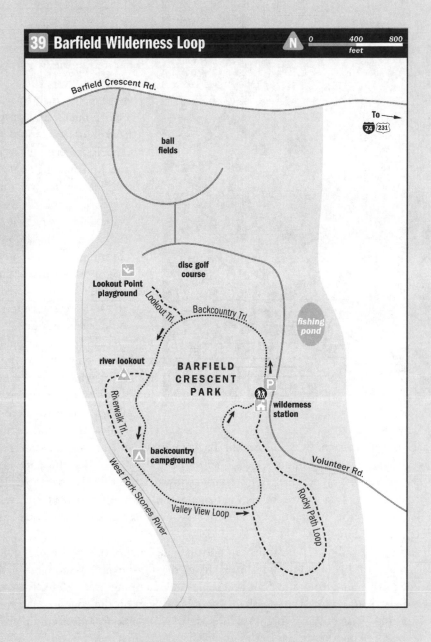

39 Barfield Wilderness Loop

N

0   400   800
feet

Barfield Crescent Rd.

To →
24 231

ball
fields

disc golf
course

Lookout Point
playground

Lookout Trl.

Backcountry Trl.

fishing
pond

river lookout

BARFIELD
CRESCENT
PARK

Riverwalk Trl.

P

wilderness
station

West Fork Stones River

backcountry
campground

Volunteer Rd.

Valley View Loop →

Rocky Path Loop

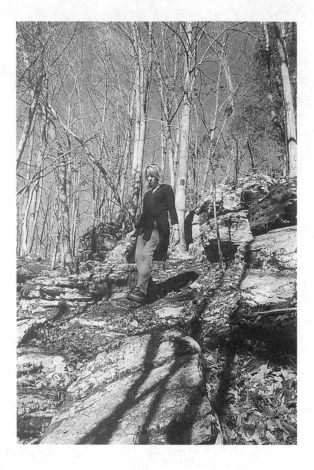

leaving the Wilderness Station, then drops alongside the West Fork Stones River, where you can enjoy a lush riparian environment and scenic rock bluffs on a footpath. The loop then picks up the Marshall Knob Trail and leaves the river for a rocky high point, passing crevasselike sinks along the way. Walk along a stone fence of unknown origin before descending among rock outcrops and sinks to return to the Wilderness Station.

Start the hike on the paved Backcountry Trail, which cuts through a hardwood forest rising above limestone out-crops. At 0.1 mile, you'll reach a trail junction. Stay left on the Backcountry Trail, as the Lookout Trail leaves right to a playground. Occasional wooden fences border the path near drop-offs. At 0.5 miles, turn right, heading toward West Fork Overlook. The paved section ends at a series of resting benches. Follow the red-blazed Riverwalk Trail down to the West Fork Stones River, which has a wide limestone shelf stretched out along it.

The Riverwalk Trail meanders in bottomland, leaving the river at 0.9 miles, and enters brushy woods. Climb away from the floodplain to soon reach the Backcountry Campground, a foot-accessible-only camping area. Here, the loop hike veers right, joining the Marshall Knob Trail. Stay on the edge of the flood-plain as the West Fork again comes into view. Walk among limestone outcrops while overlooking the stream in this especially scenic area.

Leave the river a final time, nearing a field and private property. Begin the climb toward Marshall Knob and pick up an old woods road. Reach a limestone sink and continue rising to reach a long stone fence at mile 1.6.

This fence is a subject of much speculation, as it is too high to be a livestock fence. A clue may be the second name of the high point: Marshall Knob is also known as Rebel Hill. General Braxton Bragg was a commander for the Confederacy during the Battle of Stones River. He came down this way and occupied what is now the park. From atop Rebel Hill, about where the stone fence is, Bragg could see all the way to the courthouse in downtown Murfreesboro. The Rebels signaled each other between town and Rebel Hill as they prepared to defend the Nashville Chattanooga Railroad from the Union Army. That is what makes the structure perplexing. The stone fence could have defended an advance from the south, but that was unlikely, as Bragg knew, since the Union was in Nashville to the north. Try to come up with your own theories when you hike this trail.

The Valley View Loop leaves east just past the stone fence, making a 1-mile loop. Then the trail parallels the fence and turns with it to reach a high point. Descend from Marshall Knob and head down to briefly pick up a gullied roadbed, passing more crevasselike sinks. Some of these narrow sinks are lined with ferns, which can thrive in the cooler, moister sink environment despite the drier conditions at ground level. Pass both ends of the Rocky Path Loop, then reach a low point and work among limestone to come to the Wilderness Station at mile 2.5.

NEARBY/RELATED ACTIVITIES

Barfield Crescent Park is the incarnation of the modern city park. It has the traditional ball fields and playgrounds, but it also includes a disc golf course and other paved trails for hiking and biking. The Wilderness Station offers outdoor programs led by park staff. For more information, call (615) 217-3017.

40 BRENTHAVEN BIKEWAY CONNECTOR

KEY AT-A-GLANCE INFORMATION

LENGTH: 2.4 miles

CONFIGURATION: There-and-back

DIFFICULTY: Easy

SCENERY: Riparian forests, stream

EXPOSURE: Partly shady

TRAFFIC: Busy

TRAIL SURFACE: Asphalt

HIKING TIME: 1.4 hours

ACCESS: No fees or permits

MAPS: Available at www .brentwood-tn.org

FACILITIES: Restrooms, water at Crockett Park

SPECIAL COMMENTS: The greenway is extended on both ends, adding walking distance opportunities. River Park has basketball courts. The Brentwood Library is just across the street from River Park. And Crockett Park has tennis courts, ball fields, and picnic shelters. For more information about these parks and the status of the greenway, call (615) 371-2208.

IN BRIEF

This greenway connects two parks operated by the city of Brentwood: River Park and Crockett Park. The trail traverses an attractive wooded corridor along the Little Harpeth River, which makes it one of the most attractive greenways in metro Nashville.

DESCRIPTION

I heard about this greenway from a friend of a friend. As it turns out, this connector trail between River Park on the north and Crockett Park on the south is popular with Brentwood residents—walkers, runners, and bicyclists alike. Similar to many areas of metro Nashville, the city of Brentwood is growing rapidly. However, this greenway and the adjacent parks are examples of the city planning and growing its recreational needs along with the increased population. A fine library is just across the street from the north trailhead, River Park. When designing this library, the city planners included ample green space along with extensions of the greenway, integrating the latter into the overall design rather than adding it as an afterthought.

Luckily for us, the city had some good natural terrain with which to work. It so happens that the scenic Little Harpeth River flows

GPS Trailhead Coordinates

UTM Zone (WGS84) 16S

Easting   0519140

Northing   3983310

Latitude   N 35° 59' 45.5"

Longitude   W 86° 47' 15.5"

Directions

From Exit 71 on I-65 south of downtown Nashville, take TN 253 east, Concord Road, 0.5 miles to Knox Valley Drive. Turn right on Knox Valley Drive and follow it just a short distance to River Park, on your left. Start this section of the greenway by crossing the bridge over the Little Harpeth River near the basketball courts.

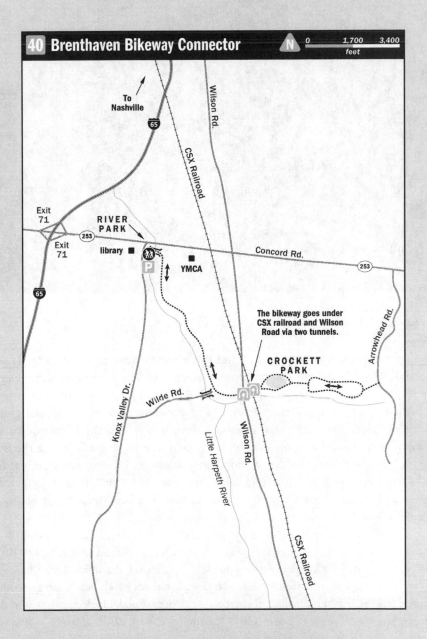

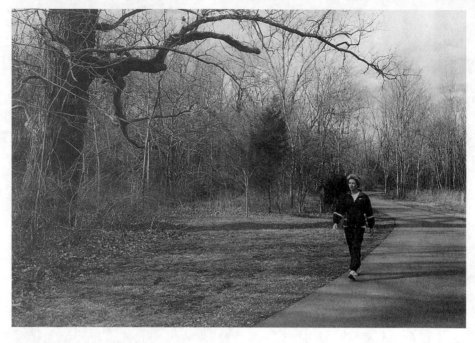

A hiker passes a massive oak tree.

through this section of Brentwood, and this river corridor made for a likely and available slice of land on which to put a greenway. The Little Harpeth River is longer than you may imagine. It actually drains 895 square miles of land, mostly in Williamson County. Soldiers from North Carolina, who received land grants for their efforts during the Revolutionary War, first settled the Brentwood area. Many plantations were in the area by the time of the Civil War. During the war, the area was pilfered of its crops and farm animals, and the homes were used as makeshift hospitals. The area languished after the Civil War but grew again after the coming of Interstate 65 in the 1960s. It has since become a major bedroom community of Nashville.

The Little Harpeth River flows adjacent to the River Park parking area. Look for the greenway bridge and begin your walk. Span the Little Harpeth River and turn south; the YMCA is off to your left. Sycamores shade the Little Harpeth River, which flows in riffles, pools, and occasional rocky shoals. During winter, houses will be visible through the trees. And occasional black-painted wooden fences, like those seen at horse farms, border the trail. Williamson County was horse country before suburbanization made its way down here, and its residents still pride themselves on this equestrian association. Plenty of horse farms still exist in rural sections of the county.

At 0.5 miles, the canopy opens overhead. A partially wooded wetland lies to the left of the trail, and to your right the Little Harpeth River has widened as it flows over a limestone slab cutting across the watercourse. The Little Harpeth had another name long ago, one that would excite anglers. In 1768, Thomas Hutchins named the river Fish Creek because he must have eaten a few meals out of this clear-green watercourse. By the 1780s, the name Harpeth began appearing on maps. It was likely derived from Big Harp and Little Harp, two highwaymen whose ilk was common in this era when Middle Tennessee was sparsely populated. Such bandits would typically lie in wait for unsuspecting travelers and rob them.

Ahead is a massive trailside oak tree with a trunk so wide that it would easily take two people together to wrap their arms around the giant. At mile 1, the trail splits. To the right, a bridge leads over the Little Harpeth River to Wikle Road and houses; this is also where the Moores Lane Greenway has been extended 0.7 miles south toward Moores Lane. The main path curves left, now alongside a feeder branch of the Little Harpeth River. A large open field is beside the trail.

Keep forward and pass through a pair of tunnels, the first tunnel passing beneath Wilson Road and the second beneath CSX Railroad tracks. You'll reach Crockett Park at mile 1.2, just beyond the tracks, and the end of this section of greenway. This large park has tennis courts, ball fields, and more. The greenway continues in Crockett Park, making a pair of small loops. And a side path leads to Arrowhead Drive. This section is not nearly as scenic as the portion along the Little Harpeth. It does, however, offer added distance for increased exercise opportunities.

The trail extends west from River Park as well, entering Concord Park and forming two loops. The trail is also being extended north across Concord Road. Stay tuned.

41 FLAT ROCK CEDAR GLADES AND BARRENS HIKE

KEY AT-A-GLANCE INFORMATION

LENGTH: 3.4 miles

CONFIGURATION: Balloon

DIFFICULTY: Moderate

SCENERY: Cedar and hardwood forest, large cedar barrens

EXPOSURE: Half shady, half sunny

TRAFFIC: You will have the trail to yourself.

TRAIL SURFACE: Rocks, dirt

HIKING TIME: 2 hours

ACCESS: No fees or permits

MAPS: Available at www.state.tn .us/environment/na/natareas/ flatrock/flatrock.pdf

FACILITIES: None

SPECIAL COMMENTS: This may be the best-preserved cedar-glade environment in Middle Tennessee.

GPS Trailhead Coordinates

UTM Zone (WGS84) 16S

Easting 0563860

Northing 3968120

Latitude N 35° 51' 25.7"

Longitude W 86° 17' 33.4"

IN BRIEF

This special area, bought and preserved by the Nature Conservancy in conjunction with the state of Tennessee, has become more special with the expansion of its trail system. Flat Rock is one of the largest intact cedar glades still remaining. The expanded loop wanders among cedar woods and along barren rock glades, grassy glades, and hardwood forest. Along the way it passes a clear alluring spring and also a sinkhole, where a creek flows into it and disappears underground.

DESCRIPTION

Flat Rock is one of Tennessee's largest intact cedar glade preserves, protecting 600 acres of the Southeast's rarest habitats. Working in conjunction with the Tennessee State Natural Areas Program, the Nature Conservancy played a large role in protecting this land, specifically known as a limestone-outcrop glade. Barren in appearance, this habitat is home to very rare plants. One flower in particular, Pyne's ground plum, is found here and at only three other known sites in the world. Pyne's ground plum was once thought to be extinct. Within this

Directions

From Exit 78B on I-24 southeast of downtown Nashville, take TN 96 east as it winds through Murfreesboro 5.6 miles to North Rutherford Boulevard. Turn right on North Rutherford Boulevard and follow it 1.3 miles to Greenland Road. Turn left on Greenland Road as it turns into Halls Mill Road, traveling a total of 3 miles to Factory Road. Turn right on Factory Road and follow it 0.9 miles to the parking area for the preserve, which will be on your right. Watch carefully for the brown sign indicating the preserve, as it is easily missed.

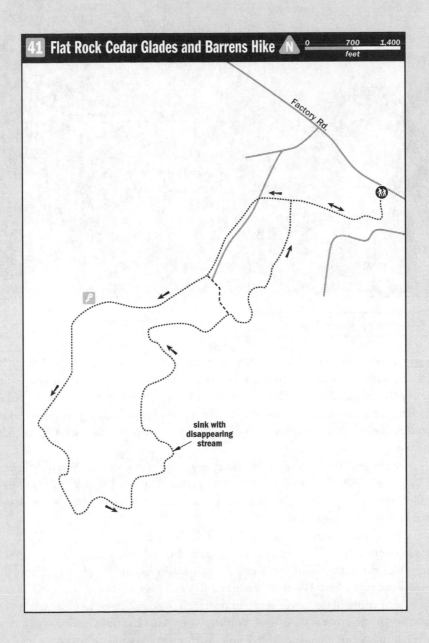

41 Flat Rock Cedar Glades and Barrens Hike

N

0   700   1,400
feet

Factory Rd.

sink with
disappearing
stream

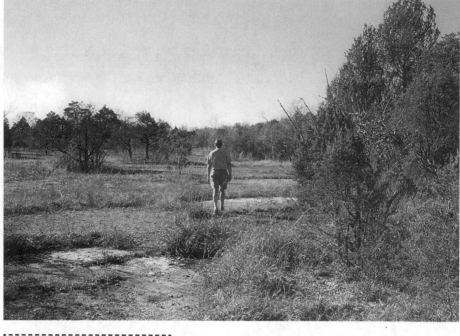

Passing through a gravelly glade

preserve are other rare plants, such as Purple prairie clover and the Sunny Bell Lily. As with other landscapes of this type, sinks, caves, and water seeps dot the seemingly dry landscape. This underground flow of water plays a large role in shaping the plants and animals that thrive in this harsh-looking country. Above-ground, wet-weather washes harbor endangered plant species such as Boykin's milkwort.

One reason the Nature Conservancy invested in this site was not only because of Pyne's ground plum and the other rare plants, but also because man had minimally impacted the site. You will see evidence of past use here, but it doesn't detract from this great hike.

This expanded path, traveling through the preserve, is one of Middle Tennessee's newer trails. Leave the parking area, shortly passing a plaque commemorating the preservation of the locale. Pass a trailside kiosk with trail maps, then enter a cedar thicket. The trail is marked by blue blazes, though you will also see occasional white blazes and—more importantly—posts tipped in blue with arrows pointing in the correct direction. Follow these posts carefully, as the path heads through many open glades. At 0.1 mile, turn right, passing behind a nearby residence. Pick up a rocky woods road along a fence line.

At 0.3 miles, you'll reach a junction; to your left is your return route. Continue forward here, climbing a hill. Flat Rock Preserve does have vertical variation, as evidenced by the views of oak-cloaked hills in the distance from the wide-open glade here. Veer left onto an old farm road, and at 0.6 miles reach a trail junction. Here, the old loop keeps forward, but the newer, blue-blazed loop turns right and heads uphill through woods, passing an old junk pile before reaching a spring at 1.0 mile. Watch as the water passes beneath the trail via a small culvert. The clear spring is to your right and emerges from a round pool about 8 feet in diameter. You can be sure that early settlers took note of this spring.

The trail continues ascending, with a rocky hill to the right, and traces an old roadbed until 1.3 miles, where it turns left and descends. Look left in the woods for the dam of an old farm pond. Along the hike you may notice where young cedars have been cut down. This is part of the glade-restoration process, which also uses prescribed burns.

At 1.5 miles, the trail winds through an open glade where old poles are stacked. The path winds in and out of small glades before reaching an area with many yucca plants at 1.9 miles. Then the trail enters a dense cedar copse and reaches a significant sinkhole at 2 miles. Here, a stream flows into the sink, briefly running in the hole before disappearing into the ground. This is indicative of the area's karst topography, which is a fancy word for holey eroded ground where water and rock interplay beneath the surface, resulting in both springs and sinks. You will undoubtedly also notice trash in the sink. Historically, settlers in glade-and-sink country filled the depressions with farm debris and trash to fill them up and stop the sinking of water from the surface. Even more elementary, the nature-made holes were good dumps. The real result was tainted water supplies wherever the water reemerged from the sink. Today, people are more aware of the interrelationship of land and water, therefore this practice is on the wane.

The trail continues through the best of what Flat Rock has to offer, but watch carefully as the trail goes where you think it won't—or shouldn't. At 2.7 miles, you'll reach the old inner loop in a large gravelly glade. At first glance, the area looks like a parking lot grown over with weeds. But these weed-looking plants are actually some of the life that is so rare in this rare habitat. The flowers that grow in this barren area are best observed from mid-August to mid-September, though other good wildflower displays are from mid-April through mid-May.

This spot is one large gravel glade, an important reason the Nature Conservancy purchased this tract. Areas known as post-oak barrens also support native grasses and endangered flowers, such as slender blazing star. The trail continues northeast, winding among more glades before completing the loop portion of the hike at 3.1 miles. Turn right here and backtrack to the trailhead.

NEARBY/RELATED ACTIVITIES

Consider combining this excursion with a trip on the Stones River Greenway of Murfreesboro or a visit to Stones River National Battlefield. Both are nearby and detailed in this book (see pages 186 and 190).

42 OLD MILL TRAIL

KEY AT-A-GLANCE INFORMATION

LENGTH: 1 mile

CONFIGURATION: Loop

DIFFICULTY: Easy

SCENERY: River, river bluff, creek, woods

EXPOSURE: Mostly shady

TRAFFIC: Some traffic on weekends, otherwise quiet

TRAIL SURFACE: Wood chips, rocks, dirt

HIKING TIME: 30 minutes

ACCESS: No fees or permits

MAPS: Available at state.tn.us/ environment/parks/gis/pdf/ printmaps/henryhorton.pdf

FACILITIES: Restrooms, water at campground; picnic table at trailhead

IN BRIEF

The Old Mill Trail traverses the most historic parcel of Henry Horton State Park. The path loops along the scenic Duck River through an area that was once the thriving hamlet of Wilhoites Mill. Experience first-hand the fading of history, as second-growth woods slowly camouflage the remains of a community that thrived in the 1800s.

DESCRIPTION

The Old Mill hike is a walk into history, heading through a community once known as Wilhoites Mill. This first white settlement in the Duck River Valley began in the late 1700s. Later, Andrew Jackson himself crossed the Duck here while establishing a road, at what was then known as Fishing Ford, on the way to the Battle of New Orleans. Later, a stage line followed Jackson's road, and a log inn was built where the state-park inn now stands. In the 1820s, the first bridge was built over the Duck at this location. This bridge and many others, including a covered bridge erected in 1838 (you can still see its rock piers), were subsequently built and swept away by floods. Around 1845, Addie Wilhoite bought the log inn. Her son John built a mill, grinding corn and grain along the Duck River. It was around

GPS Trailhead Coordinates

UTM Zone (WGS84) 16S

Easting   0533720

Northing   3995490

Latitude   N 36° 6' 17.9"

Longitude W 86° 37' 31.2"

Directions ————————→

From Exit 46 on I-65 south of Nashville, head east on TN 99 13 miles to US 31A. Turn right on 31A and follow it south a short piece to the Henry Horton State Park. Look left for a parking area just before 31A bridges the Duck River. This left turn is just across from the right turn into the state-park campground.

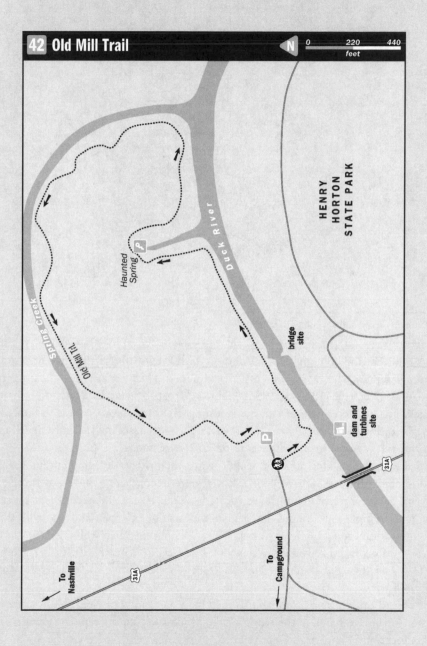

42 Old Mill Trail

N

0   220   440
feet

Duck River

HENRY HORTON STATE PARK

Haunted Spring

Spring Creek

Old Mill Trl.

bridge site

dam and turbines site

31A

To Nashville

31A

To Campground

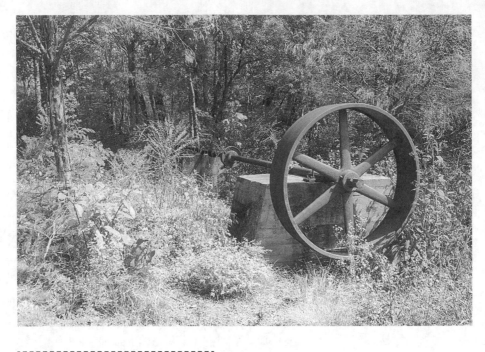

Remnants of old mill powering operation

this mill that the community of Wilhoites Mill grew. John Wilhoite married and had a daughter who married Henry Horton, later a U.S. senator and the governor of Tennessee from 1927 to 1933. Henry Horton returned to his home on the Duck, but he died just one year after ending his term as governor. His son John operated the mill until 1959, when the site was purchased by the state of Tennessee for the establishment of the state park you see today.

Leave the parking area and walk toward the bridge, descending on a path of wood chips. Immediately to your left is a large iron wheel, which was turned by a long belt, connected to turbines located on the river. This setup kept most of the mill on higher ground, as the original mill had been wiped out in a 1902 flood during which the Duck River rose 47 feet in 11 hours! Keep walking down to the river, and on its bank you'll see the rock-filled cedar cribs that held the turbines. A low dam diverted water through the turbines that drove the gears and turned the millstones.

Head upriver just a short bit to the bridge site on your right. Here, rock relics of the bridge pinch in the Duck River, which then shoots rapidly downstream. This location is known as Fishing Ford, the spot where Andrew Jackson crossed the Duck.

Continue forward in a riparian area, where wildflowers bloom throughout the summer. In other places, cedars thrive on the edge of limestone bluffs over which the trail passes. Side trails lead down to flat limestone outcrops along the river. Anglers may be seen down here, lazing away the day as the green Duck River flows downstream to meet the Buffalo River, which meets the Tennessee River. The trail turns away from the river as it passes over a few ravines via wooden bridges. The path is circling around Haunted Spring. Legend has it that a washwoman for the Horton family had her baby in a cloth sling as she was laundering at the spring. Her baby got away from her, fell in the river, and was never found despite a massive search. Folks got to thinking the spring must be haunted to take away a baby so rapidly.

You'll briefly come near the Duck River before turning upstream along Spring Creek, which is heavily grown up with beard cane along its edges. This rocky watercourse has bluffs of its own and may nearly dry out in summer and fall. Overhead, a young cedar thicket is reclaiming the village of Wilhoite Mills. Keep heading up along the creek. Imagine a post office, scales, and a store that were once here, and a blacksmith shop that stood across the creek. Turn away from the creek along a wetland. Pass under a straight old woods road that was undoubtedly part of the village and emerge in the trail parking area.

NEARBY/RELATED ACTIVITIES

Henry Horton State Park offers not only hiking but also excellent tent camping, while the Duck River offers good fishing and family canoeing. A canoe livery very near the state park rents canoes and offers shuttle service. For more information, call (931) 364-2222 or visit **www.tnstateparks.com**.

43 OLD STONE FORT LOOP

KEY AT-A-GLANCE INFORMATION

LENGTH: 2.6 miles

CONFIGURATION: Loop

DIFFICULTY: Moderate

SCENERY: High river bluffs, narrow rock ridge, riverside bottomland, waterfalls

EXPOSURE: Mostly shady

TRAFFIC: Moderate to busy

TRAIL SURFACE: Wood chips, leaves, rocks

HIKING TIME: 2 hours

ACCESS: No fees or permits

MAPS: Old Stone Fort Archaeological State Park Area Map at park office

FACILITIES: Restrooms, water at museum

SPECIAL COMMENTS: Visit the museum before you go on your hike

IN BRIEF

This is one of Middle Tennessee's better hikes. You'll make a loop between the forks of the Duck River, circling around a 2,000-year-old stone wall built by ancient Native Americans. Other features include several large waterfalls, rock bluffs, and remnants of mill dams. An interpretive guide and state-park museum enhance the experience.

DESCRIPTION

The narrow spit of land between the forks of the Duck River is the setting for this hike, which melds Native American history with the natural beauty of this fine state park. After leaving the museum, this hike circles an ancient Native American enclosure marked by a stone wall. Pass along Step Falls and the bluffs of the Little Duck River before dropping into the Moat, an abandoned river channel. Climb along the narrow rocky ridge of the Backbone, before dropping back down to the water's edge to again meet the Little Duck. Follow it to the confluence with the main Duck River. Climb past more of the stone wall and waterfalls of the Duck, along with old mills, before completing the loop.

After visiting the museum, begin your hike on the Wall Trail. Stay to your left, looking at

GPS Trailhead Coordinates

UTM Zone (WGS84) 16S

Easting   0533720

Northing   3927130

Latitude   N 35° 29' 10.4"

Longitude   W 86° 6' 8.0"

Directions

From Nashville, take I-24 east to Exit 111, Manchester. Head west on TN 55 0.8 miles, then turn right on US 41, heading north. Keep forward on US 41 1.7 miles and turn left into Old Stone Fort State Park. Continue forward in the park, following signs to the Old Stone Fort and parking near the museum. The hike starts near the museum.

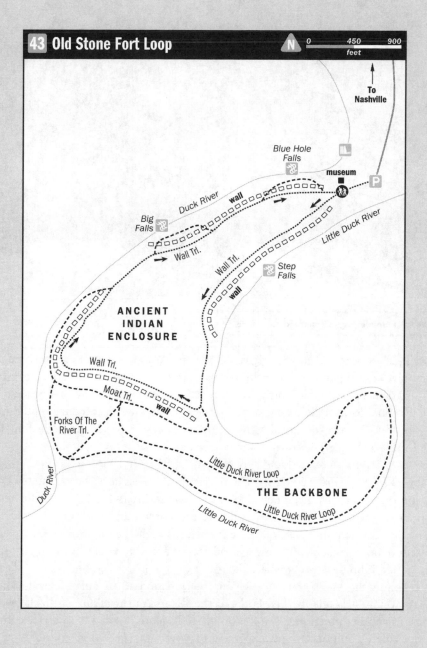

43 **Old Stone Fort Loop**

N

0   450   900
feet

To
Nashville

Blue Hole
Falls

museum

P

Duck River   wall

Big
Falls

Wall Trl.

Wall Trl.

Step
Falls

Little Duck River

wall

ANCIENT
INDIAN
ENCLOSURE

Wall Trl.

Moat Trl.

wall

Forks Of The
River Trl.

Little Duck River Loop

Duck River

THE BACKBONE

Little Duck River Loop

Little Duck River

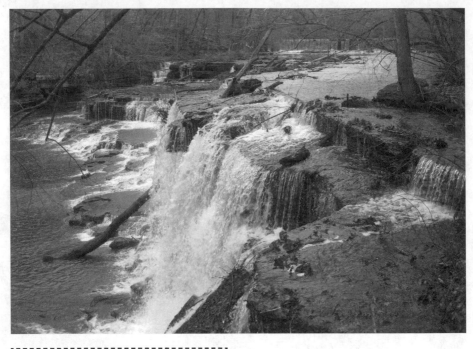

Big Falls tumbles over a fractured rock ledge.

the 50-acre open field to your right. Because few artifacts were found, archaeologists have concluded that this enclosure was a ceremonial place and not a defensive or a settlement location. Shortly, you'll reach a wooden walkway that heads over the wall and down to Step Falls on the Little Duck below. Visit the falls and return via another boardwalk, returning inside the old wall. Cruise alongside the bluffs of the Little Duck, peering down toward the water.

At 0.5 miles, you'll reach a concrete marker from 1966, which is used as a mapping point by archaeologists. The trail splits just past here. Turn left, descending on the River Channel Trail, also known as the Moat Trail. Veer right into a former riverbed of the Duck River, before the watercourse bursts through a narrow ridge formed long before Native Americans built the Old Stone Fort, which was developed over a 400-year period, from approximately AD 1 to AD 400. Beech and tulip trees grow where the water once ran.

Follow the Moat Trail to reach another junction at 0.7 miles. Turn left here on the yellow-triangle-marked Forks of the River Trail, walking just a short distance to another junction. Turn left on the red square marked "Little Duck River Loop," then climb onto the Backbone, a narrow rock ridge cloaked in mountain laurel. The Backbone widens a bit before the trail descends to the banks of the Little Duck River. This area will be rich with wildflowers in spring. Walk downstream alongside the Little Duck amid lush woods. Bluffs form a rampart on the far side of the stream.

The bottomland gives way, as a hill on your right and the river on the left hem in the trail. The rocky, rooty track reaches another junction at mile 1.8. Stay to your left, now on the yellow-triangle-marked Forks of the River Trail, and reach the confluence of the Duck and Little Duck rivers. Stand there and lament not having a fishing pole, then climb away to meet another junction. Stay to your left here on the Red, Green, and Yellow Trail Access. Rise to meet the Wall Trail again. Stay left, again, heading up the Duck River on a high bluff. Time has rendered the stone wall less noticeable here.

You'll soon reach a side trail leading left down to Big Falls, a massive cascade dropping over a rock face into a huge pool. A rock shelf stands beside the falls. Be very careful because the rocks are slippery around here. Look back away from the falls and you'll see large stone blocks, remnants of some mill operation. The path splits again—stay closer to the river—leading over a boardwalk and passing a more intact mill operation. This mill, the Whitman Mill, was built in 1852. Later, the Hickerson and Wooten Mill provided pulp for newspapers across Tennessee and the South, creating an entire community around the operation.

The final stop is the side trail to Blue Hole Falls, which is longer and wider than Big Falls. Ahead is a dam built in 1963, before this was a state park. Shortly, return to the museum and grab one last view from the observation platform above the museum. The questions you may have about the Old Stone Fort will probably require another visit to the museum after your hike.

NEARBY/RELATED ACTIVITIES

Old Stone Fort State Archaeological Park is one of Tennessee's most unsung destinations. Consider complementing your hike with a camping trip here. For more information, visit **www.tnstateparks.com.**

44 SHORT SPRINGS STATE NATURAL AREA HIKE

 KEY AT-A-GLANCE INFORMATION

LENGTH: 2.9 miles

CONFIGURATION: Loop with spur trails

DIFFICULTY: Moderate

SCENERY: Hardwood forest, waterfalls

EXPOSURE: Shady

TRAFFIC: Moderate

TRAIL SURFACE: Leaves, rocks

HIKING TIME: 2.5 hours

ACCESS: No fees or permits

MAPS: Available at www.tennessee .gov/environment/na/natareas/ shortspr/shortspr.pdf

FACILITIES: None

SPECIAL COMMENTS: Hike every trail at this state natural area.

GPS Trailhead Coordinates

UTM Zone (WGS84) 16S

Easting   0575000

Northing 3918400

Latitude N 35° 24' 28.6"

Longitude W 86° 10' 26.8"

IN BRIEF

This woodland in Coffee County is one of the best hiking destinations in Middle Tennessee. A well-developed trail system passes by clear streams that form waterfalls as they drop off of the Eastern Highland Rim into the Nashville Basin. Dry, oak-cloaked ridges stand tall between these deep valleys where the water flows.

DESCRIPTION

Get here early to hike all the trails. This 420-acre state natural area includes rich woods, forest ravines, low cascades, springs, and big waterfalls, one of which I think should be in Tennessee's Top Ten Waterfalls List.

Thomas Busby saw power in the flowing water and built a mill here in the 1820s. After the mill closed, people began to believe that the translucent waters of these streams possessed healing powers, and locals tried to attract tourists to the area. Today, the area is managed cooperatively by the city of

Directions

From Nashville, head east on I-24 to Exit 111, Manchester. From there, take TN 55 west 5 miles to Belmont Road. There will be a sign here that reads, "TVA Normandy Dam." Turn right on Belmont Road and follow it 1.2 miles to Rutledge Falls Drive. Turn left on Rutledge Falls Drive. Follow Rutledge Falls Drive 1.4 miles to reach a three-way stop. Turn right here, still on Rutledge Falls Drive. Follow Rutledge Falls Drive 2 miles to Short Springs Road. (Short Springs Grocery is on this corner.) Turn left on Short Springs Road and follow it 0.8 miles to reach trailhead parking, on your left beneath a huge water tower. The trail starts on the far side of the road.

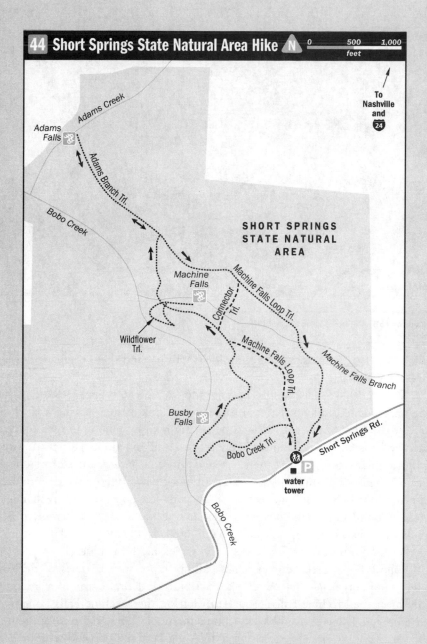

44 Short Springs State Natural Area Hike

N

0   500   1,000
        feet

To
Nashville
and
24

Adams Creek

Adams
Falls

Adams Branch Trl.

Bobo Creek

SHORT SPRINGS
STATE NATURAL
AREA

Machine
Falls

Machine Falls Loop Trl.

Connector
Trl.

Wildflower
Trl.

Machine Falls Loop Trl.

Machine Falls Branch

Busby
Falls

Bobo Creek Trl.

Short Springs Rd.

water
tower

P

Bobo Creek

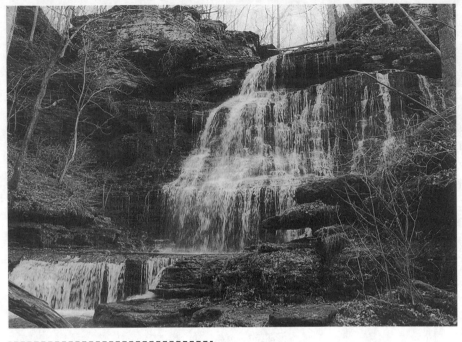

Machine Falls stairsteps over a rock bluff.

Tullahoma, the Tennessee Valley Authority (TVA), and the Tennessee Division of Natural Heritage.

The trailhead is hard to miss because the words "Short Springs State Natural Area" are painted in giant letters on the water tank at the parking area. Leave here, cross Short Springs Road, and begin the hike by joining the white-blazed Machine Falls Loop Trail. Immediately reach a trail junction; the return portion of the loop leaves right. Stay left, passing through an area of storm-damaged trees, and reach a second junction and trail kiosk where there may be trail maps. Take the blue-blazed Bobo Creek Trail to your left and descend, reaching the concrete foundation of the former Scout camp at 0.4 miles. Soon come to Bobo Creek, with its numerous cascades, highlighted by the two-tiered Busby Falls. Another loop trail leading left across Bobo Creek has been added here.

Follow Bobo Creek downstream, gaining more stream views of the rock-walled mini-gorge. Parallel the creek on a bluff and circle around a hollow to again meet the Machine Falls Loop. Turn left on the Machine Falls Loop Trail, and soon you'll meet the red-blazed Connector Trail leading right, to shortcut the loop. Straddle the ridgeline, passing a TVA marker, and descend steep steps to reach Machine Falls Branch and a trail junction at mile 1.1. Turn right and head upstream directly alongside Machine Falls Branch, heading for Machine Falls. The trail traces a narrow rock shelf along the crystal-clear stream.

Machine Falls drops 60 feet over a moss-and-rock face. (Adventurous hikers can make the short trip to the rock house to the left of the falls.) Backtrack to the trail junction and take the Wildflower Loop. Two rare state-listed flowers call Short Springs home: nestronia and the broad-leaved bunchflower. The Wildflower Trail circles bottomland at the confluence of Machine Falls Branch and Bobo Creek.

Return to the junction again (rock-hop across Machine Falls Branch) back onto the white-blazed Machine Falls Loop. Ascend away from the streams and go toward the oak ridgeline to make another junction. Turn left here, following the Adams Creek Trail. This orange-blazed path undulates in and out of forested ravines roughly paralleling Bobo Creek before descending to Adams Creek and a sign indicating Adams Falls at mile 1.8.

Backtrack to again reach the Machine Falls Loop at mile 2.2. Ahead, Machine Falls is audible before the Machine Falls Loop intersects the Connector Trail, which crosses Machine Falls Branch via a footbridge above Machine Falls. Keep forward, up Machine Falls Branch, to rock-hop the stream at mile 2.6. Ascend to a hardwood forest and pass beneath a power line. Stay with the white blazes to soon complete the loop.

45 STONES RIVER BATTLEFIELD LOOP

KEY AT-A-GLANCE INFORMATION

LENGTH: 3.6 miles

CONFIGURATION: Loop

DIFFICULTY: Easy

SCENERY: Forest and field

EXPOSURE: Half sunny, half shady

TRAFFIC: Moderate, especially last half of trail

TRAIL SURFACE: Dirt, rocks, pavement, gravel, grass

HIKING TIME: 2.8 hours

ACCESS: No fees or permits

MAPS: Available at www.nps.gov/stri

FACILITIES: Restrooms, water, picnic area at visitor center

IN BRIEF

This loop hike traverses many of the interesting sites at Stones River National Battlefield. See earthworks, cannon emplacements, memorials, and cemeteries interspersed into an attractive environment of woods, cedar glades, and fields. Though the path is called the Five Mile Trail, it is only 3.6 miles long. Combine this hike with a trip to the battlefield visitor center and a short auto tour to familiarize yourself with an important chapter of Middle Tennessee history.

DESCRIPTION

This loop hike travels throughout the preserved portion of the battlefield where the Union and the Confederacy battled for control of the road and railroad connecting Nashville with states to the south. These lines were important for supplying troops of both sides. The Union strategy west of the Appalachian Mountains was to control the Mississippi River and drive a wedge into the Confederacy along the railroads of Tennessee and Georgia. With this second objective in mind, Union General William Rosecrans left his winter quarters in Nashville and headed from Murfreesboro, where the Confederacy's Braxton Bragg was stationed.

GPS Trailhead Coordinates

UTM Zone (WGS84) 16S

Easting 0550980

Northing 3970700

Latitude N 35° 52' 51.5"

Longitude W 86° 26' 5.9"

Directions

From I-24 southeast of downtown Nashville, take Exit 74B to TN 840 east. From 840 east, take Exit 55A, Murfreesboro, and head south on US 41/70 south 2 miles to Thompson Lane. Turn right on Thompson Lane, then travel 0.3 miles and turn left to access Old Nashville Highway. Turn left on Old Nashville Highway, follow it 0.7 miles, and turn left into the visitor center. The Five Mile Trail starts at the picnic area near the visitor center.

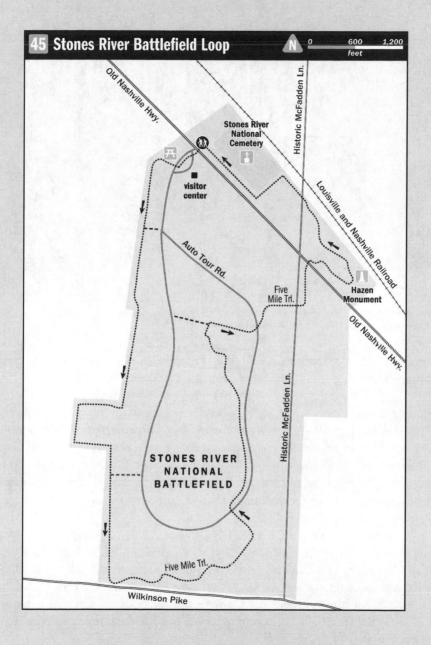

45 Stones River Battlefield Loop

N

0   600   1,200
feet

Old Nashville Hwy.

Historic McFadden Ln.

Stones River
National
Cemetery

Louisville and Nashville Railroad

visitor
center

Auto Tour Rd.

Five
Mile Trl.

Hazen
Monument

Old Nashville Hwy.

Historic McFadden Ln.

STONES RIVER
NATIONAL
BATTLEFIELD

Five Mile Trl.

Wilkinson Pike

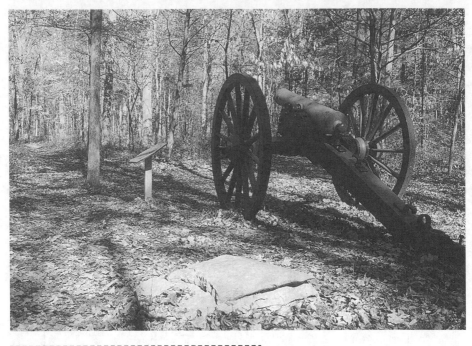

A cannon marks the position of the Alabama Battery.

With forces totaling more than 80,000 men combined, the two armies clashed during a three-day period, starting December 31, 1862.

The Confederates struck first, but their offensive was stopped. The two armies remained entrenched on New Year's Day, fighting little. But January 2, 1863, was a bloody day in American history, as a Confederate assault was pushed back by heavy cannon fire. Later, Braxton Bragg withdrew toward Chattanooga. The tactically indecisive battle resulted in more than 13,000 casualties. Today, you can walk amid much of the battle site, contemplating what happened on those fateful winter days. I recommend making this loop in winter to gain a better perspective of those troubled years.

The Five Mile Trail leaves the picnic area as a mowed path entering a cedar thicket. You'll soon turn left, passing a sign indicating Federal entrenchments. Then head south along the battlefield boundary, marked by a wire fence. Occasional limestone outcrops break the gravel path. At 0.3 miles, a trail leads left to the location on the auto-tour road, where the Feds put up a line of defense to stop the initial Rebel assault. Continue forward in a cedar forest, passing a second trail leading left to the road.

The Five Mile Trail skirts around the battlefield boundary, passing a military park-survey marker before reaching a cannon representing the position of the Alabama Battery. Another side trail leads left to the auto-tour road. The Five Mile Trail keeps forward, passing a marker indicating the site of the Blanton log house, just outside the park. Turn west here, nearing a road before turning into an area of cedars and rock outcrops. A side trail leads right to a sedate field, once the site of fighting so fierce it became known as the Slaughter Pens. The Five Mile Trail leads left, past damaged cannons that were left as the Union retreated in haste over the rugged terrain. Follow a paved path to the auto-tour road and turn right, tracing the road.

At 2 miles, keep an eye peeled for the footpath leading left into the woods. Continue forward, as side trails split left from the footpath. Soon open onto a field bordered by a split-rail fence. The visitor center is across the field. Turn right here, opening onto the auto-tour road at stop No. 1. Cross the auto-tour road, picking up Parsons Battery, a paved path that passes cannon emplacements on your left. Soon you'll reach the crumbling pavement of McFadden's Lane. Turn left on this historic road, now closed to automobiles, and follow it among fields to Old Nashville Highway just ahead.

Turn right on Nashville Highway, passing by a tollhouse site. Cross Old Nashville Highway at the white stripes painted on the road, and pass through the split-rail fence on the far side of the road. Turn right, heading on a mowed path toward Hazens Monument. Take the paved path among large trees to enter the monument, which was erected in 1863 and is the oldest Civil War monument in existence. After Bragg retreated, Union men stayed in Murfreesboro for six months. While here, they interred their dead and built this memorial.

As you face the monument, look left for a path heading into the Round Forest, a site of major fighting. This location lies between what the battle was fought for—the railroad to your right and Nashville Pike to your left. Cross back over McFadden's Lane and keep forward, passing a marker noting where one of Rosecrans's aids was killed. Soon reach a stone wall, across which is the Stones River National Cemetery. Only Union soldiers, nearly half of whom are unknown, were buried in this still-active burial place. Walk along the wall back toward Old Nashville Highway and parallel the road, crossing Old Nashville Highway one last time to reach the park visitor center, completing the loop.

NEARBY/RELATED ACTIVITIES

Stones River National Battlefield has a visitor center that offers a slide show and informative displays about this battle, in particular, and the Civil War, in general. Take time to enjoy the slide show and consider taking the auto tour as well. For more information, visit **www.nps.gov/stri**.

46 STONES RIVER GREENWAY OF MURFREESBORO

KEY AT-A-GLANCE INFORMATION

LENGTH: 6 miles round-trip

CONFIGURATION: There-and-back

DIFFICULTY: Moderate

SCENERY: River valley, fort earthworks

EXPOSURE: Partly shady

TRAFFIC: Fairly busy, but path is wide

TRAIL SURFACE: Asphalt

HIKING TIME: 3 hours

ACCESS: No fees or permits

MAPS: Available at www.murfreesborotn.gov

FACILITIES: Restrooms, water at General Bragg trailhead, halfway along trail

SPECIAL COMMENTS: Path also connects to Lytle Creek Greenway and Stones River National Battlefield

GPS Trailhead Coordinates

UTM Zone (WGS84) 16S

Easting   0553017

Northing   3967527

Latitude   N 35° 51' 8.0"

Longitude   W 86° 24' 45.2"

IN BRIEF

The Stones River Greenway offers hikers a chance to enjoy both human and natural history in Murfreesboro. This paved path links earthworks and important sites from the Civil War's Battle of Stones River as it courses alongside the attractive Stones River.

DESCRIPTION

This greenway forms the link between various parcels of preserved portions of the Stones River National Battlefield. But this trail is not just about Civil War history, it's also about recreation and appealing natural scenery along the Stones River as it flows through Murfreesboro. The nearly level trail leaves the old Fortress Rosecrans, then heads north, passing sites such as Braxton Bragg's Headquarters before ending near the old McFadden farm.

Start the walk at Fortress Rosecrans. What you see at the trailhead is but one side of what once was the largest enclosed earthen fortification built during the Civil War. The Union occupied Murfreesboro after the Battle of Stones River, which they won, but the main Union supply post was at faraway Louisville, Kentucky. General William Rosecrans ordered a fortified supply depot built here, so he could continue south toward Chattanooga and beyond. Rosecrans was following the Union strategy of driving a wedge through the Confederacy, ultimately leading to General Sherman's "March to the Sea." What you see today

Directions ———————————▶

From Exit 78 on I-24 southeast of downtown Nashville, take TN 96 east 1.3 miles to Golf Lane. Turn left on Golf Lane and follow the signs to Stones River Greenway.

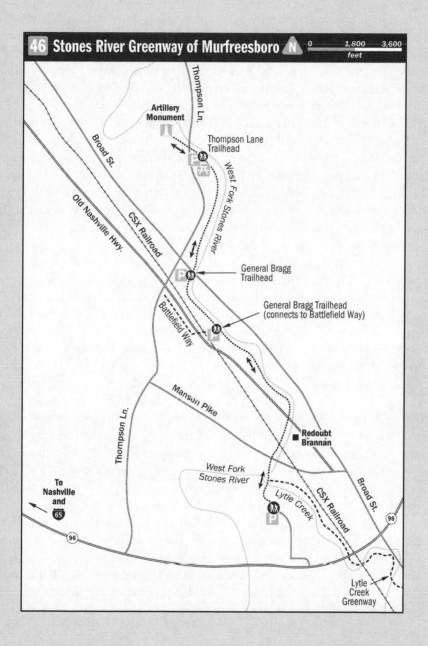

46 Stones River Greenway of Murfreesboro

0   1,800   3,600
feet

Thompson Ln.

Artillery
Monument

Thompson Lane
Trailhead

Broad St.

West Fork Stones River

Old Nashville Hwy.

CSX Railroad

General Bragg
Trailhead

General Bragg Trailhead
(connects to Battlefield Way)

Battlefield Way

Manson Pike

Thompson Ln.

Redoubt
Brannan

West Fork
Stones River

To
Nashville
and
65

Lytle Creek

CSX Railroad

Broad St.

96

96

Lytle
Creek
Greenway

are the earthworks remaining from that supply depot. Walkways lead up to the earthworks and are enhanced with interpretive information.

Leave the parking area and head north along the paved and landscaped greenway. Fortress Rosecrans is off to your right. Soon you'll reach the iron trestle bridge over Lytle Creek. Here, the Lytle Creek Greenway goes to the right, and the Stones River Greenway goes to the left, staying atop a floodplain and crossing the Stones River. The Stones River Greenway is now on the west bank of the Stones River, where it will remain for the rest of the hike.

Look for an old mill dam, over which the Stones crashes and splashes. Pass the Manson Pike trailhead, then walk underneath the old Nashville and Chattanooga Railroad—the rail line that prompted the Battle of Stones River. Reach the side trail to Redoubt Brannon at 0.7 miles. This trail leads left up to College Street and crosses the College Street Bridge back over the Stones River to reach the only remaining of four interior earthwork forts in Fortress Rosecrans. The College Street Bridge is where the Nashville Turnpike Bridge, which once was the road connecting Nashville and Chattanooga, stood.

Keep forward along the Stones River, passing a canoe launch for this popular paddling and fishing river. Silver maple, hackberry, and other moisture-loving trees line the watercourse. Signs identify tree specimens along the greenway. The canopy is often open overhead. Reach the side trail leading left to the General Bragg Headquarters Site and trailhead at mile 1.6. This is the most developed trailhead and is also where the spur greenway leads along College Street to reach Stones River National Battlefield near the Hazen Monument.

Here, the Stones River Greenway leaves the floodplain for a rocky riverside bluff, offering a different river perspective. Pass the Broad Street trailhead at mile 2. Beyond here, the greenway becomes less used, as there are fewer access points. Shortly reach Harker's Crossing, the site where Union soldiers crossed the Stones, scouting and running directly into Confederate positions. This skirmish gave the Union important information on strategic Confederate emplacements.

The greenway is now back along the river, which flows in alternating riffles and pools. Continue forward as the greenway becomes busy again near the Thompson Lane trailhead, which is reached at mile 3. You can choose to turn around here, or continue forward 0.2 miles farther, passing a canoe launch and beneath Thompson Lane to reach the McFadden Farm Site and the Artillery Monument. Here, Union soldiers repulsed a costly Confederate assault. From atop this hill it is easy to see how difficult it must have been for the Rebels to cross the Stones River and climb the hill where Union cannons were firing away with deadly accuracy.

NEARBY/RELATED ACTIVITIES

The Stones River Greenway is just one path in a greenway network of Murfreesboro. The Lytle Creek Greenway departs from the same trailhead as the Stones River Greenway, and the Battlefield Greenway connects the Stones River Greenway to the battlefield site.

TWIN FORKS TRAIL 47

IN BRIEF

This hike makes a loop around the East Fork Recreation Area on the upper reaches of Percy Priest Lake. East Fork refers to the East Fork Stones River. The trail curves along the river, which nearly turns back along itself. Enjoy river bluffs and bottomlands in this slice of Rutherford County.

DESCRIPTION

This is just one segment of a 20-mile trail that winds along the banks of the East Fork and West Fork Stones River, connecting Nice's Mill Recreation Area on the upper West Fork Stones River and the upper East Fork Stones River near Walter Hill Dam Picnic Area. Trail users can pick up the Twin Forks Trail at the above areas, as well as at the West Fork Recreation Area. The U.S. Army Corps of Engineers has an excellent map that will help steer you around Percy Priest Lake.

The East Fork Recreation Area is roughly in the middle of the Twin Forks Trail. Though the path was built with equestrians in mind, hikers are welcome and frequently use the section around East Fork Recreation Area. This is a good place to get a taste of the Twin Forks

KEY AT-A-GLANCE INFORMATION

LENGTH: 1.5 miles
CONFIGURATION: Loop
DIFFICULTY: Easy
SCENERY: Cedar bluffs, river bottom forest
EXPOSURE: Mostly shady
TRAFFIC: Moderate, busier on warm weekends
TRAIL SURFACE: Dirt, rocks
HIKING TIME: 1 hour
ACCESS: No fees or permits
MAPS: Obtain map and interpretive guide online at www.lrn.usace.army.mil/op/jpp/rec
FACILITIES: Restrooms, water at East Fork Picnic Area

Directions

From I-24 southeast of downtown Nashville, take Exit 74B to TN 840 east. Follow 840 east to Exit 57, Sulphur Springs Road. Turn left on Sulphur Springs Road and follow it 0.6 miles to Buckeye Valley Road. Turn right on Buckeye Valley Road and follow it 2.9 miles to East Fork Recreation Area. Turn left into East Fork Recreation Area and follow the road 0.1 mile to the first right turn into a large parking area. As you are facing the water at the boat ramp, take the trail to your left.

GPS Trailhead Coordinates

UTM Zone (WGS84) 16S
Easting   0549870
Northing   3981830
Latitude   N 35° 58' 52.2"
Longitude   W 86° 26' 48.4"

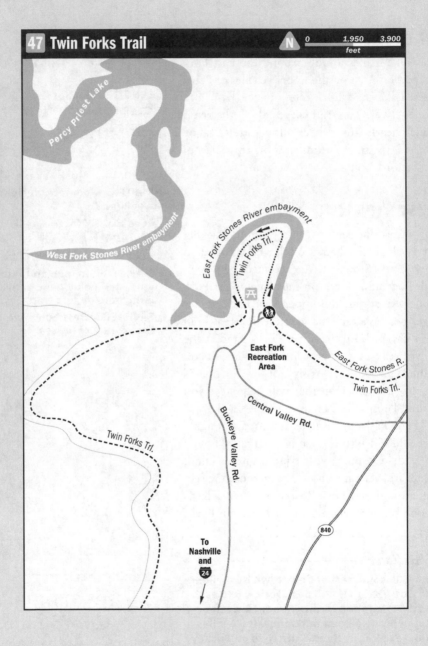

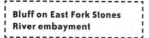

Bluff on East Fork Stones
River embayment

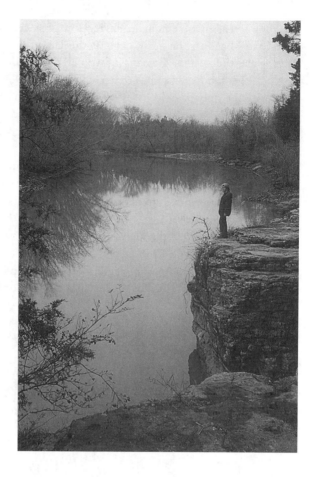

Trail, as you can make a loop hike out of it because the East Fork Stones River makes such an acute bend as to nearly double back on itself.

Start the hike by leaving the large parking area near the boat ramp; a little sign with a horse on it marks the path. The Twin Forks Trail also leaves from the other side of the parking area. If you start heading toward TN 840, you are going the wrong way. If you are going the right way, enter young brushy wood and reach some high limestone bluffs overlooking the East Fork Stones River. At this point the river is dammed but still has a narrow channel and does exhibit flow. Little side trails lead to the cedar-studded bluffs and overlook points.

The East Fork embayment widens as you keep downriver. The bluffs give way, and the Twin Forks Trail drifts down to a bottomland hardwood forest. The path can be wet here, as it circles among the sycamore and maple trees. At 0.6 miles, a side trail leads right, to the river embayment. Bluffs stand tall on the far side of the East Fork.

Straddle the shaded and wooded margin between a field that covers the middle of the big river bend you are circling. This field is sown with crops to attract wildlife. In fact, bird boxes have been placed in the bottomlands for further wildlife enhancement. At mile 1.2, rise a bit from the bottomland into brushy young woodland. Soon you'll reach the East Fork Picnic Area, which has tables, grills, water, and restrooms. Big trees scattered in the grassy picnic area indicate that this may have been a homestead.

Recreation areas such as this were not always included in the long history of the Army Corps of Engineers, which was mostly about improving waterways for commerce. Involvement in navigation projects by the Army Corps of Engineers dates back to the early days of the United States, when rivers and waterways were the primary means of travel and trade. As the lands west of the original 13 states began to be settled, rivers became even more important, because they were the only practical way of getting through the country's vast forests and mountains. Henry Clay of Kentucky lobbied for federal assistance in maintaining the navigability of such waters. Others thought it wasn't the job of the federal government. The Supreme Court settled it, ruling that the commerce clause of the Constitution enabled the Feds to not only regulate navigation and commerce but also to make improvements in navigable waters. That decision gave birth to the Corps and its mission to maintain harbors, rivers, waterways, and, ultimately, trails and picnic areas.

Continue forward through the picnic area to reach the crumbling remnants of an asphalt road. The Twin Forks Trail turns right here. You, however, turn left and follow the old road past a picnic shelter to the picnic parking area. Turn right at the parking area, and follow the road a bit to soon reach the trail parking area on your left.

NEARBY/RELATED ACTIVITIES

The East Fork Recreation Area has a boat ramp, picnic tables, shelters, grills, and an added segment of the Twin Forks Trail. The picnic area is closed in the cold season. For more information, call (615) 889-1975.

WILD TURKEY TRAIL   **48**

IN BRIEF

Henry Horton State Park's longest trail, Wild Turkey Trail, makes a loop through a cedar–oak–hickory forest that is fast reclaiming former farmland. You will see old fence lines and woods roads. Its low hills divided by intermittent streambeds make for some vertical variation as the path passes beside limestone outcrops and sinkholes. The mix of old fields and young woods makes for good wildlife habitat, not only for wild turkeys but also for deer.

DESCRIPTION

As we see more and more of Middle Tennessee getting eaten up by strip malls, roads, and subdivisions, it is heartening to see a slice of land return to its natural state. Such is the case in Henry Horton State Park, located just south of the Duck River. The state of Tennessee owns the parkland, which it purchased from John Horton in the late 1950s. His father, Henry Horton, was a U.S. senator and later governor of Tennessee from 1927 to 1933. Henry Horton married into the Wilhoite clan, which owned and operated a farm and mill on the banks of the Duck River for more than a century. The community of Wilhoites Mill grew around this area, and there was once a

KEY AT-A-GLANCE INFORMATION

LENGTH: 2.5 miles

CONFIGURATION: Loop

DIFFICULTY: Easy

SCENERY: Rolling, mostly forested country

EXPOSURE: Mostly shady

TRAFFIC: Moderate

TRAIL SURFACE: Wood chips, dirt, rocks

HIKING TIME: 1 hour

ACCESS: No fees or permits

MAPS: Available at www.state .tn.us/environment/parks/ HenryHorton

FACILITIES: None at trailhead

SPECIAL COMMENTS: Trail may be closed during very occasional archery events at park archery range

---

Directions

From Exit 46 on I-65 south of Nashville, head east on TN 99 13 miles to US 31A. Turn right on 31A and follow it south to Henry Horton State Park. After you pass over the Duck River on 31A, keep forward 1 mile to Warner Road. Turn left on Warner Road and drive 0.2 miles to the trailhead, which will be on your right, near a park-maintenance building across from Riverside Road.

GPS Trailhead Coordinates

UTM Zone (WGS84) 16S

Easting 0528150

Northing 3937600

Latitude N 35° 35' 0.3"

Longitude W 86° 41' 20.9"

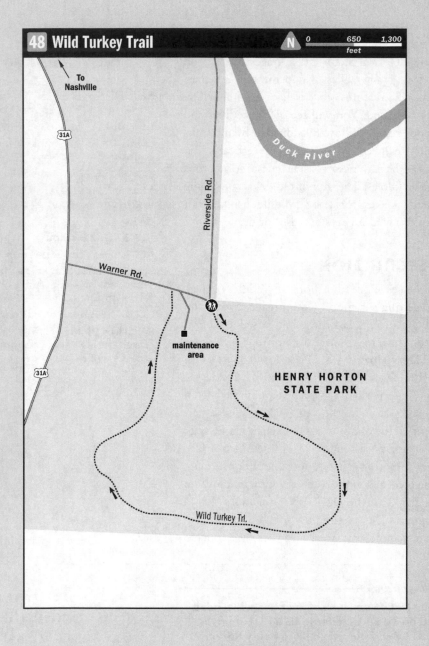

48 Wild Turkey Trail

N

0   650   1,300
feet

To
Nashville

31A

Duck River

Riverside Rd.

Warner Rd.

maintenance
area

HENRY HORTON
STATE PARK

31A

Wild Turkey Trl.

post office, blacksmith shop, and general store. But times have changed in Duck River country since Henry Horton's day. You will get a firsthand glimpse of those changes while walking through what once was open farm country. The state park is letting the area regenerate at its own pace, in its own time.

Leave the Wild Turkey trailhead, heading south, and descend into a hickory, maple, and cedar forest, complemented with oak trees. Cedar trees love the limestone underpinnings of the soil here. Often the limestone emerges from the ground as it does on many of the moss-covered outcrops you will see. The orange-blazed trail leads to a seasonal streambed that is more richly grown up than the thinner soil adjacent to it. In these depressions you are likely to find deer feeding or turkeys scratching. Turn away from the seasonal streambed and come to your first farm evidence—an old wire fence. Notice that the wooden posts of the fence are made of cedar, which resists rot well, assuring that these posts will be standing for a long time. Keep forward, looking right through the woods for a small pond. This was a farm pond meant for domesticated critters such as cattle or horses. These days, forest creatures like raccoons, foxes, skunks, and more make use of it. Look around for tracks on the edge of the pond.

The trail opens ahead and comes to a fast-disappearing clearing. Here, an old grassy farm road runs perpendicular to the trail. Look around at the edges of the clearing and see the brush and young trees growing here. These edges make for good wildlife feeding grounds as well. In not too many years, this clearing will completely disappear. Meander through shallow depressions and low hills, keeping an eye out for a sinkhole to the right of the trail. Here, a break in the limestone has allowed water to seep to a less-resistant layer of rock and worn it away, causing the surface to collapse and forming a depression with no outlet for water. The lands around the state park and the Duck River basin are laced with sinkholes from which water runs underground and reemerges elsewhere. That is why some local farm ponds that stay full should seemingly dry up but don't—they are fed from underground. In contrast, some areas, like this sinkhole, won't hold water no matter what. Look for a couple of other sinkholes along the trail.

Curve around the state-park boundary now heading north. Look for shallow straight-line depressions in the forest that indicate other old farm roads. Returning north, the trail traces an old woods road that parallels a wire-and-wood fence. Meander over more low swales to emerge onto Warner Road. Turn right and walk a short distance back to the trailhead.

NEARBY/RELATED ACTIVITIES

Henry Horton State Park offers not only hiking but also excellent tent camping. The nearby Duck River offers fishing and canoeing and has a fine picnic area along its banks. A canoe livery very near the state park rents canoes and offers shuttle service. For more information, call (931) 364-2222 or visit **www .tnstateparks.com.**

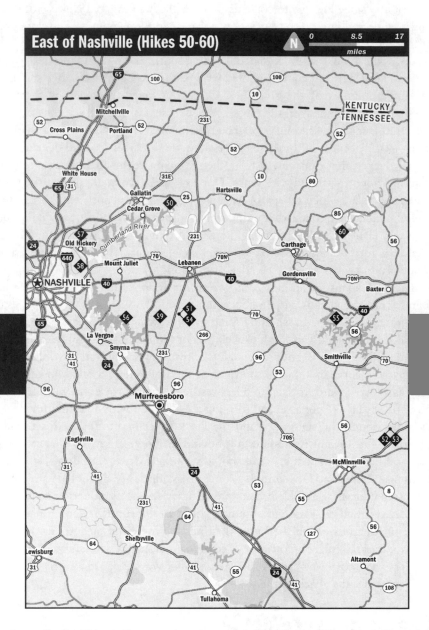

East of Nashville (Hikes 50-60)

0   8.5   17
miles
N

KENTUCKY
TENNESSEE

Mitchellville
Cross Plains
Portland
White House
Gallatin
Cedar Grove
Hartsville
Old Hickory
Cumberland River
Carthage
Mount Juliet
Lebanon
Gordonsville
Baxter
NASHVILLE
La Vergne
Smyrna
Smithville
Murfreesboro
Eagleville
McMinnville
Shelbyville
Lewisburg
Altamont
Tullahoma

49 Bearwaller Gap Hiking Trail............... 202
50 Bledsoe Creek State Park Loop 206
51 Cedar Woods Trail........................ 210
52 Collins River Nature Trail 214
53 Eagle Trail................................. 218
54 Hidden Springs Trail...................... 222

55 John C. Clayborn Millennium Trail 226
56 Jones Mill Trail........................... 230
57 Old Hickory Trail 233
58 Peeler Park Greenway 237
59 Vesta Glade Trail 241
60 Wilderness Trail 245

EAST
INCLUDING GALLATIN, HENDERSONVILLE, LEBANON, AND MOUNT JULIET

49 BEARWALLER GAP HIKING TRAIL

KEY AT-A-GLANCE INFORMATION

LENGTH: 11.2 miles

CONFIGURATION: There-and-back

DIFFICULTY: Difficult

SCENERY: Wooded lakeshore and bluffs, numerous streams

EXPOSURE: Mostly shady

TRAFFIC: Busy during warm-weather weekends

TRAIL SURFACE: Leaves, dirt, rocks

HIKING TIME: 6 hours

ACCESS: No fees or permits

MAPS: Available at www.lrn.usace .army.mil/op/cor/rec/bearwaller .htm

FACILITIES: Restrooms, water at day-use area during warm season

SPECIAL COMMENTS: A backcountry campsite is located along the trail.

IN BRIEF

This is one of the finest paths in Middle Tennessee. It extends along the wooded and rugged shoreline of Cordell Hull Lake for more than 5 miles, passing waterfalls, old homesites, and rocky overlooks. It will challenge hardy hikers as it climbs and descends numerous times. Bring your stamina and ample time with you.

DESCRIPTION

Let's face it, some hikes are more rewarding than others. And the Bearwaller Gap Hiking Trail is one of the most rewarding hikes in Middle Tennessee. Why? It travels a considerable distance—5.6 miles one way. Although it offers an old spring and other evidence of human habitation, it passes numerous natural features: rock gardens, overlooks, wet-weather waterfalls, and wildflowers in season. And it is physically challenging, traversing many ups and downs along the shoreline of Cordell Hull Lake. You can even backpack here because the trail has a designated backcountry campsite. Hikers can halve their distance, if confined by time and effort—the trail has parking areas at

GPS Trailhead Coordinates

UTM Zone (WGS84) 16S

Easting   0535919

Northing   3995737

Latitude   N 36° 6' 26.3"

Longitude   W 86° 36' 3.3"

Directions ⟶

From Exit 258 on Interstate 40 east of downtown Nashville, take TN 53 north 4 miles, and continue forward as the road changes into TN 25 west. Keep forward 6 more miles to reach TN 80. Turn right on TN 80 north and follow it 2.5 miles to TN 85. Turn right on TN 85 east, and follow it 3.6 miles to Defeated Creek Recreation Area. Turn right and follow the recreation-area road 1.4 miles to a parking area on the right just before the campground-entrance station. In winter, you must park over by the marina, beyond the campground-entrance station.

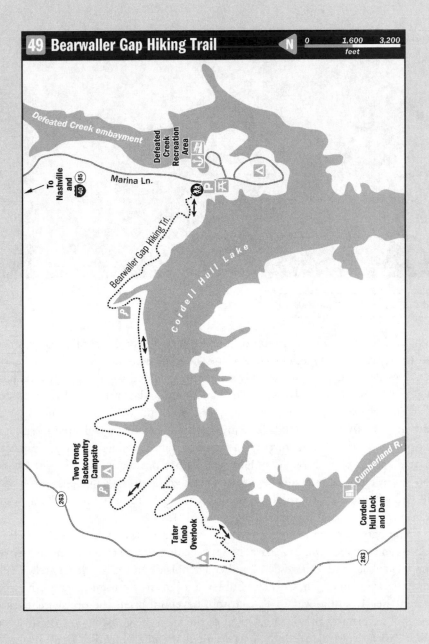

49 Bearwaller Gap Hiking Trail

N

0   1,600   3,200
feet

Defeated Creek embayment

Defeated Creek Recreation Area

Marina Ln.

To Nashville and 40 85

Bearwaller Gap Hiking Trl.

Cordell Hull Lake

Two Prong Backcountry Campsite

263

Tater Knob Overlook

Cumberland R.

Cordell Hull Lock and Dam

263

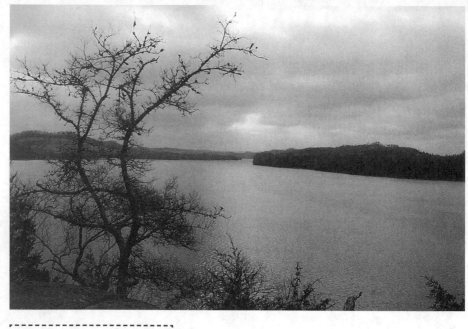

Cloudy day at Cordell Hull Lake

both ends, giving you the option of going either 5.6 or 11.2 miles. Be apprised that the Tater Knob Overlook trailhead is gated in winter.

This designated national recreation trail is named for the practice of bears "wallering" in moist shady places during summer. Alas, no bears live in Middle Tennessee these days, though you may see deer and wild turkeys on this trail. Start the hike by leaving the U.S. Army Corps of Engineers Defeated Creek Recreation Area and passing through a wooden fence beside the large trail sign. Immediately ramble through young brush before passing a second sign. Cross a wooden bridge and immediately enter a rock garden. Look just past the bridge, and you will see a small "window" in a rock to the right of the trail. Wind, water, and time have created this interesting geologic feature.

The path is blazed along its entire length in yellow, white, and sometimes red. Ascend through the rock garden, appreciating other strangely shaped stones, then switchback into a hardwood-and-cedar hillside to reach a level area. Cruise along the wooded bench. Cordell Hull Lake looms to your left through the trees, as it will nearly all the way to Tater Knob. Level out briefly before switchbacking downhill to turn toward an embayment of the lake; the going is slow on this steep slope. Pass a dry streambed, then a perennial stream, which has small waterfalls both above and below the trail. Curve around the embayment, passing a couple more streambeds. You can now see down this embayment into the main lake. Look for a spring on your right in brushy woods. It has a concrete block catch basin, and just above the basin is the rocked-in springhead. A homesite was undoubtedly in the vicinity.

Continue forward and enter a grassy area at mile 1.5. Stay to the left, with the brown sign and arrow indicating the correct direction. (More of these signs are placed at strategic points along the trail.) The Bearwaller Gap Hiking Trail now enters young woods and veers to the right, away from the lake. You'll reach a rock bluff that offers great southerly views of the dammed Cumberland River. Keep ascending on a narrow ridgeline to top out on a knob. Cordell Hull Lake is 400 feet below. Descend from the knob and pass two more rock-bluff overlooks before crossing an intermittent streambed.

Begin to skirt an embayment known as Two Prong. Curve around Ashopper Hollow, stepping over the streambed that creates the hollow, and come alongside a stone fence in this formerly settled area. Curve around the second prong of Two Prong and reach Two Prong Backcountry Campsite at mile 3. This area has flat spots for camping, in addition to a covered spring, fire pits, a covered camping shelter, a picnic table, and an outhouse. Day hikers cutting their trip short can shoot for Two Prong as a turnaround point, making for a 6-mile there-and-back.

The trail climbs a wide roadbed to top out at mile 3.3, near a gate. Turn left here and make an easy and glorious walk along a southbound level ridgeline. Look for narrow, knife-edge sinkholes on the ridge. This easy walking soon ends, as the path travels past some odd-looking stacked-rock piles. Curve off the ridgeline, heading downhill to cross a rocky streambed at mile 4.1. Work around the small embayment with mossy walls of stone reaching to the waterline of Cordell Hull Lake. Shortly you'll pass an old homesite, where ivy has grown wild and crosses the trail.

Beyond this point, the path ascends to come alongside a shoreline bluff. Cordell Hull Dam and other nearby bluffs are visible in the distance, and the lake lies far below. Just as you seem to near the dam, the Bearwaller Gap Hiking Trail veers abruptly right, away from the dam, and climbs toward Tater Knob. Reach the overlook restrooms at mile 5.5. Keep ascending past the restrooms to top out on a developed overlook. From here, hikers are rewarded with a sweeping panorama of Cordell Hull Lake, the Cumberland River, and the hill country through which it flows. From May through September, hikers can leave a shuttle car here. However, call ahead to make sure the overlook is open. Here are the directions to Tater Knob Overlook: From Exit 258 on Interstate 40 east of downtown Nashville, take TN 53 north 4 miles. Keep forward as the road changes into TN 25 west 2.6 miles to reach TN 263 north. Turn right on TN 263 and follow it 3.6 miles to the overlook.

NEARBY/RELATED ACTIVITIES

Defeated Creek Recreation Area has a campground, a marina, a picnic area, a playground, and a swim beach. For more information, call (615) 735-1034.

50 BLEDSOE CREEK STATE PARK LOOP

KEY AT-A-GLANCE INFORMATION

LENGTH: 3.1 miles

CONFIGURATION: Loop

DIFFICULTY: Easy to moderate

SCENERY: Lakeside, forest

EXPOSURE: Mostly shady

TRAFFIC: Busy during summer camping season

TRAIL SURFACE: Leaves, rocks

HIKING TIME: 1.8 hours

ACCESS: No fees or permits

MAPS: Available at www.state .tn.us/environment/parks/ BledsoeCreek/images/Bledsoe.jpg

FACILITIES: Restrooms, water at park office

SPECIAL COMMENTS: Bledsoe Creek State Park offers camping and water sports such as boating, fishing, and swimming. Picnic areas and playgrounds appeal to day visitors. For more information, visit www.tnstateparks.com.

IN BRIEF

This loop hike traverses the perimeter of Bledsoe Creek State Park. Located near Gallatin, the park borders Old Hickory Lake. The trail offers lakeside walking, in addition to some hilltop walking through prime deer and wild-turkey habitat.

DESCRIPTION

Bledsoe Creek is a small state park, and this loop makes the most of the scenic terrain included in this 164-acre preserve. Part of the scenery may well be wild turkeys. I don't know if it is just my luck, but wild turkey sightings have been part of every visit. It seems the turkeys are used to human contact, as they slowly but surely amble on after seeing people.

The beginning portion of the hike travels along paved all-access trails before picking up the natural-terrain Shoreline Trail. This path lives up to its name, as it traces the margin of land beside Old Hickory Lake. The loop then takes you to the High Ridge Trail, which passes a homesite before climbing away from the shore and traversing a ridgeline 250 feet above Old Hickory Lake. The High Ridge Trail then connects to the Big Oak Trail, which

GPS Trailhead Coordinates

UTM Zone (WGS84) 16S

Easting 0557760

Northing 4025730

Latitude   N 36° 22' 36.1"

Longitude W 86° 21' 22.3"

Directions

From Exit 95 on I-65 north of downtown Nashville, take TN 386 east 9.3 miles to merge onto US 31E north. Continue forward on US 31E north 7 miles to TN 25 east. Turn right on TN 25 east and follow it 5.3 miles to Zieglers Fort Road. Follow Zieglers Fort Road for 1.2 miles to Bledsoe Creek State Park. Enter the park and leave your car near the park-entrance station. The hike starts on a paved path on the right, just beyond the entrance station.

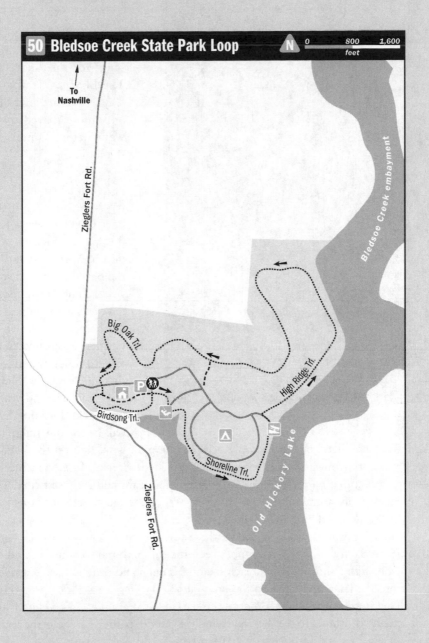

50 Bledsoe Creek State Park Loop

N

0   800   1,600
feet

To
Nashville

Zieglers Fort Rd.

Bledsoe Creek embayment

Big Oak Trl.

High Ridge Trl.

Birdsong Trl.

Shoreline Trl.

Old Hickory Lake

Zieglers Fort Rd.

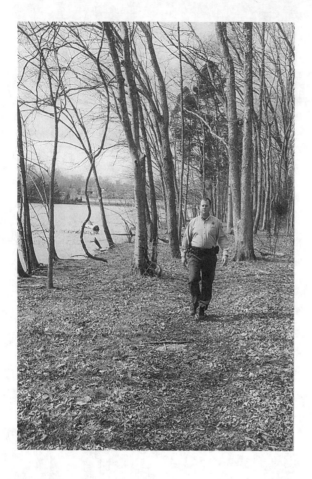

curves past another homesite before dropping to the shoreline. The Big Oak Trail gives way to the Birdsong Trail and more paved pathways before completing the loop.

The first part of the loop can be confusing, so pay attention. Start the paved path to the left of the park office as you face it. Walk forward on the paved path, and soon you'll come to a four-way paved trail junction. Veer left here, and soon you'll reach a playground. Walk toward the water and then pick up the Shoreline Trail, marked with a sign. Old Hickory Lake will be to your right. The lake looks small here, but that is only because the park is located on the Bledsoe Creek arm of the long and large impoundment. Bledsoe Creek is located in Sumner County, once a rich hunting ground for Native Americans and early settlers due to the abundance of natural salt licks in the area. Wildlife is still abundant in this state park: deer, turkey, rabbits, and even coyotes make Bledsoe Creek their home.

Watch for waterfowl as you take the Shoreline Trail, curving as the shore curves. Straddle the wooded margin between the campground to your left and the lake to your right. Shortly, you'll reach the boat launch and fishing dock. Turn left, away from the lake, and head up the boat-launch parking area. Pick up the High Ridge Trail in the upper-right corner of the parking area at mile 1. The High Ridge Trail actually continues to parallel the shoreline, but the path is far above the water. Trace an old roadbed through a mixed hardwood and cedar forest, then descend toward Old Hickory Lake. Keep an eye open for an old stone fence and level land to your left, marking a forgotten homesite. Of course, the folks who lived here looked down on a flowing Bledsoe Creek instead of the lake embayment.

Span a ravine via wooden footbridge, then climb a bluffline. Old Hickory Lake is still to your right, and soon you'll drop back to the lakeside. The High Ridge Trail just can't make up its mind to stay high or low. However, it does offer open views of Bledsoe Creek embayment. Finally, the High Ridge Trail makes up for its indecisiveness and climbs directly up the ridgeline with the help of wooden steps. A resting bench at the top of the hill looks appealing after that climb.

Soon you'll be walking along the park border, marked by a stone-and-wire fence. Skirt the border atop the ridgeline, topping out on a knob. Walk through young forest and you'll reach a trail junction at mile 2.1. Continue forward, as a side trail leaves left toward the campground. You are now on the Big Oak Trail, which soon slips off the ridgeline to the right, crossing a small spring branch on a pair of footbridges. An intact stone fence stands to the right. Climb away from this rich ravine into a cedar thicket. The campground office is visible to your left, but don't shortcut the loop—don't even think about it. Make one last climb of a hill, then descend to another stream, which is crossed on a bridge.

Reach and cross the main park road to enter a cedar thicket in a flat, now back on paved pathway. This is the Birdsong Nature Trail. Soon you'll reach a junction: stay right here and cruise along a creek before curving past the park ball field. This flat is a wildflower haven in spring. Continue forward at the final paved trail junction and complete your loop. This final area may be confusing, but the park office is very near and can be reached in a matter of a few minutes no matter which paved paths you use.

51 CEDAR WOODS TRAIL

KEY AT-A-GLANCE INFORMATION

LENGTH: 2 miles
CONFIGURATION: Loop
DIFFICULTY: Easy
SCENERY: Cedar and hardwood forest
EXPOSURE: Shady
TRAFFIC: Busy on weekends
TRAIL SURFACE: Dirt, rocks
HIKING TIME: 1 hour
ACCESS: No fees or permits required
MAPS: Cedars of Lebanon State Park and Forest Trail Map, available at visitor center
FACILITIES: Restrooms, water at visitor center; picnic area at trailhead

IN BRIEF

This loop hike shows off the trees for which Cedars of Lebanon State Park was named. The trail passes through cedar woods but also penetrates hardwood forests on some of the state park's more hilly terrain, though none of the climbs are tiresome. Exposed rock gardens—areas with bleached limestone eroded into interesting shapes—punctuate the woods. The trail also passes numerous sinkholes of different sizes.

DESCRIPTION

The trail circles the northwestern section of Cedars of Lebanon State Park, a refuge that has become more important as metro Nashville pushes ever outward. What was quiet countryside on the outskirts of sleepy Lebanon has become dotted with more and more homes.

Americans receiving land grants for their service during the Revolutionary War originally settled this area of Wilson County. When they arrived, these veterans found the land cloaked in vast cedar forests. These stands of cedar reminded them of the cedar trees of Lebanon referenced in the Bible and gave rise to the town's name. The settlers were determined to carve out a life in the cedars and

GPS Trailhead Coordinates

UTM Zone (WGS84) 16S
Easting   0560780
Northing   3993780
Latitude   N 36° 5' 19.7"
Longitude W 86° 19' 30.4"

Directions

From Exit 238 on I-40 near Lebanon, head south on US 231 6 miles to the state-park entrance, which will be on your left. Enter the park, get a trail map at the visitor center, then keep forward a short piece to reach Picnic Shelter No. 1 on your right, which is 0.8 miles from the park entrance. The Cedar Forest Trail starts on the left side of the road, opposite the picnic shelter.

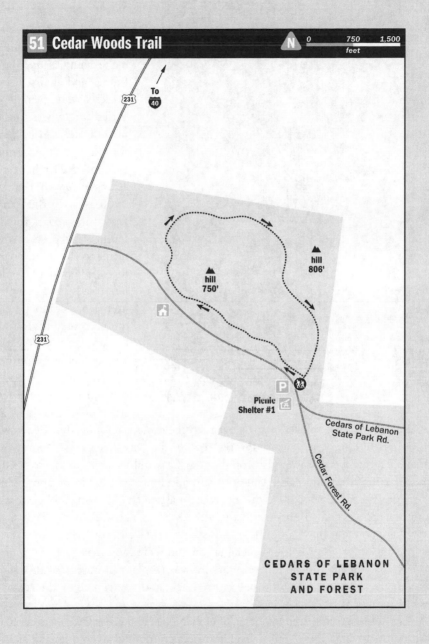

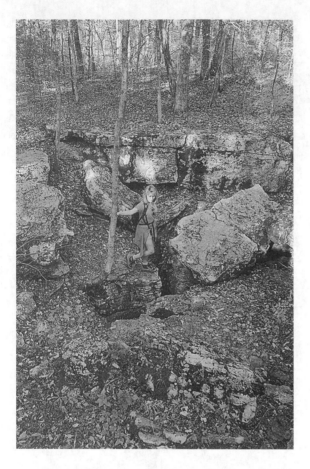

Sink next to the Cedar Woods Trail

used the trees on their farms for heating, and to make shingles and build frames and chairs. Forest pockets were cleared for agriculture where the soil was thickest. Still, cedar was king of the county. Commercial timber operations came in the late 1800s, and they harvested the cedars for different purposes than farmers—for road boarding, telephone poles, fence rails, and pencils— items that could be sold in mass quantity. Cedar has always been the preferred material for pencils because its wood is soft. In fact, Cedar Key, off Florida's Gulf Coast, was denuded for the sake of pencils in much the same fashion as this area was.

After the harvest, farms sprung up in the vast clearings. More than 60 small farms were scattered throughout what would later become the 9,000 acres of state forest and park. The poor soil and limestone outcrops upon which cedars grow were terrible for growing crops; massive tree-clearing and poor agricultural practices led to erosion of the already marginal soil. In the 1930s, the federal government purchased these subsistence farms and turned the area into a demonstration project for forest reclamation and recreation management. One of the first assignments of the federal workers was to plant hundreds of thousands of cedar trees. Today, the forest has grown back, and you can enjoy the renewed woodland on this trail.

Leave the parking area by Picnic Shelter No. 1, and cross Cedar Forest Road to reach the Cedar Forest Trail. Turn left onto a crumbling paved road and ascend. Turn left off the roadbed onto a singletrack footpath. At 0.2 miles, reach the actual loop portion of the trail. Turn right here, skirt the state-park border, and stairstep a moderate hill. Cruise alongside a rampart of rock on the hillside. A close look at the rampart will reveal subtle eroded shapes of rock carved over eons. Turn upward, cutting through the rampart to top out on a hill at 0.7 miles. The thicker soils atop this hill allow for the growth of hardwoods instead of cedars, creating more biodiversity. The trail turns left, gently drops down the hill, and begins to pass beside sinks and rock outcrops scattered beneath a forest of oak and maple. Curve around, passing a deep sink on your left. You can safely peer inside the hole here. Ahead, Cedar Forest Road is off in the distance to your right.

The trail twists and turns in a rock garden, so it is easy to see why the Works Progress Administration (WPA) of the 1930s used stone as its material of choice to construct the park buildings. The park lodge, picnic shelters, and other structures were built of native stone during this time. The impressive work of the WPA led to these buildings being added to the National Register of Historic Places.

Watch for a narrow deep sink just beside the trail on the right. Descend, then climb a bit to reach the end of the loop. Backtrack 0.2 miles on the crumbling asphalt road and complete the hike.

NEARBY/RELATED ACTIVITIES

Cedars of Lebanon State Park and Forest has more than hiking trails. It offers a good campground, picnic areas, picnic shelters, a lodge, and cabins. For more information, visit **www.tnstateparks.com.**

52 COLLINS RIVER NATURE TRAIL

KEY AT-A-GLANCE INFORMATION

LENGTH: 3 miles
CONFIGURATION: Loop
DIFFICULTY: Easy
SCENERY: Hardwood forest, big rivers
EXPOSURE: Nearly all shady
TRAFFIC: Moderate, quiet during week
TRAIL SURFACE: Leaves, dirt
HIKING TIME: 1.7 hours
ACCESS: No fees or permits required
MAPS: Available at www.state.tn .us/environment/parks/Rock Island/map.pdf
FACILITIES: Restrooms, water at park office

IN BRIEF

This trail is not a nature trail in the classic sense. It has no interpretive signs. However, it does circle the attractive peninsula between the Collins and Caney Fork rivers. Water is never far away, and a practiced eye will discern old homesites scattered in the woods about this Tennessee state park trail.

DESCRIPTION

There are many ways to get to Rock Island State Park. However, none of them are easy. So relax, make an unhurried drive from Nashville, and enjoy a full day or more at this scenic gem of a getaway. Collins River Nature Trail may be the hook to get here, but you will see there is more to behold than just this path. Swimming, boating, nature study, and camping may bring you back for more adventures. Eagle Trail, also profiled in this book, provides additional walking opportunities.

Because Collins River Nature Trail is just across the road from a powerhouse, it is not surprising that the path starts in an open field beneath power lines. These power lines are connected to the Great Falls powerhouse, which is fed by the Great Falls Dam. This dam

GPS Trailhead Coordinates

UTM Zone (WGS 84) 16S
Easting   0623440
Northing 3962890
Latitude N 35° 48' 14.7"
Longitude W 85° 38' 2.3"

Directions

From Exit 239A (Watertown) on I-40 east of downtown Nashville, take US 70 for 34 miles to TN 56 south in Smithville. Turn right on TN 56 south and follow it 9 miles to TN 287. Turn left on TN 287 north and follow it 10.6 miles, passing the main Rock Island State Park entrance on your left at 10.1 miles. Collins River Nature Trail is on the right on TN 287, across the road from the Great Falls Dam Powerhouse, 0.5 miles past the main park entrance.

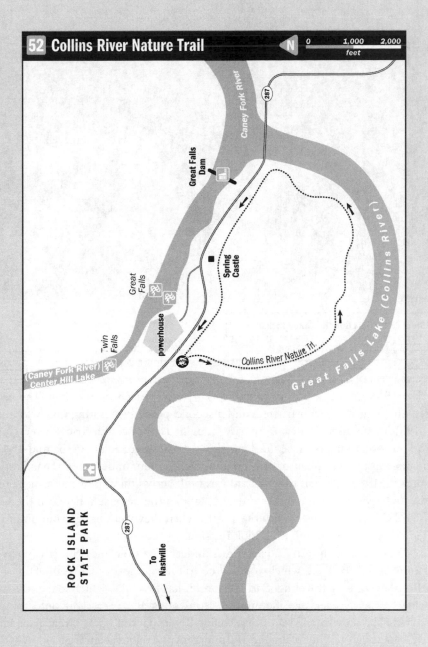

52 Collins River Nature Trail

N

0   1,000   2,000
feet

Caney Fork River

287

Great Falls Dam

Spring Castle

Great Falls

powerhouse

Twin Falls

Collins River Nature Trl.

Great Falls Lake (Collins River)

(Caney Fork River)
Center Hill Lake

ROCK ISLAND STATE PARK

287

To Nashville

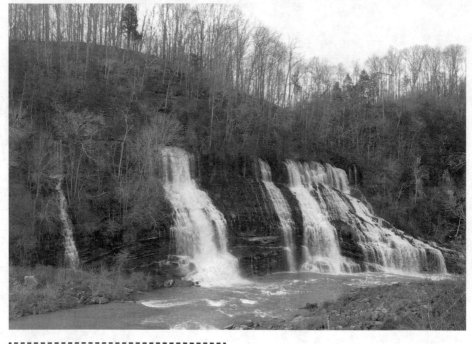

Great Falls spills into the Caney Fork River.

was one of the Volunteer State's earliest hydroelectric projects. The Tennessee Electric Power Company began constructing the dam in 1915 and completed it by late 1916. A one-unit powerhouse was erected adjacent to the dam. Ten years later, the dam was reconstructed, and a second power-generating unit was built. In 1939, Tennessee Valley Authority bought Tennessee Electric Power Company—a good thing, because the dam required extensive repairs in the mid-1940s. The dam and power plant have been in use since then, undergoing rehabilitation in the late 1980s. At that time, a road was built across the top of the dam. Before TVA took over the dam, homesteaders inhabited the peninsula between the Collins and Caney Fork rivers until the 1940s, when they were bought out and relocated. When you walk the trail, look for signs of these inhabitants.

Park at the open trailhead and cross under the power lines. Shortly, you will pick up an old roadbed, which you will be following most of the trail. This wide path makes for easy traveling. Furthermore, it has few hills, which makes the trail doable by nearly everyone. Soon enter the woods and veer right onto the old roadbed. The narrow ribbon of the Collins River, backed up as Great Falls Lake at this point, lies to your right and will stay on your right the entire loop. A short-leaf pine–and-oak forest shades the trail.

Pass under a power line, also emanating from Great Falls powerhouse, and encounter a patch of yucca plants with stalklike leaves. The folks who once lived along this old dirt road likely planted the ancestors of these plants. A second smaller power line opens the landscape and allows views of the Collins River. The trail continues turning with the Collins River toward the Caney Fork, and the TN 287 bridge comes into view. The path veers right, off the roadbed, near Great Falls Dam, which is visible to the right through the trees.

After you backtrack over the old roadbed, keep your eyes open for the small Cunningham Cemetery to the left of the trail. The graves here have newer stones. The most prominent of the stones is that of John Cunningham, a veteran of the War of 1812. A dug well is near the graves, to the right of them as you face them from the trail. Stones have been laid in a circle down the well to keep its walls from caving in, but the bottom of the well has filled in. This is part of a homesite. I can only wonder which was here first—the graves or the well. It is unusual to have a well so close to a graveyard.

The next trail section reveals more homesite evidence. The forest is evenly aged. Small, level flats are scattered in the woods. Look for metal relics, such as old washtubs. Spring Castle, located toward Caney Fork River, fed water to these homesteads. This circular building, still visible today from TN 287, captured water flowing off the bluff below and pumped it up to these residences. Great Falls Cotton Mill is located near the Spring Castle. This square brick building is pinched in between TN 287 and Caney Fork River. It used waterpower to gin cotton but was in operation only a decade before floodwaters destroyed the waterwheel in the early 1900s. At this point, Collins River Nature Trail leaves the woods and emerges into a clearing broken by a large oak tree. The powerhouse is visible across the road. Make a short walk through the grass to complete the loop.

NEARBY/RELATED ACTIVITIES

Rock Island State Park has an excellent campground, playgrounds, game courts, a boat launch, and other trails. Be sure to see Twin Falls and Great Falls while you are here. They are visible from the road over Great Falls Dam. For more information, visit **www.tnstateparks.com**.

53 EAGLE TRAIL

KEY AT-A-GLANCE INFORMATION

LENGTH: 1.7 miles

CONFIGURATION: There-and-back

DIFFICULTY: Moderate

SCENERY: Riverside woods, bluffs, water galore

EXPOSURE: Mostly shady

TRAFFIC: Busy on warm weekends

TRAIL SURFACE: Dirt, rocks

HIKING TIME: 1 hour

ACCESS: No fees or permits required

MAPS: Available at www.state.tn .us/environment/parks/Rock Island/map.pdf

FACILITIES: Restrooms, water at trailhead

GPS Trailhead Coordinates

UTM Zone (WGS84) 16S

Easting 0624060

Northing 3962816

Latitude N 35° 48' 12.2"

Longitude W 85° 37' 37.5"

IN BRIEF

The sound of falling water is ever-present along this path that traverses the gorge of the Caney Fork River. Located below Great Falls Dam at Rock Island State Park, the trail connects two of the park's picnic areas and includes a rock scramble and river access at one end.

DESCRIPTION

This path packs a punch (and a half) into its short length set along a rugged portion of the Caney Fork River. You will pass by smaller waterfalls to end near one of the state's most famous falls. How this falling water came to be is an unusual story.

In 1915, Tennessee Electric Power Company dammed the Caney Fork River, creating Great Falls Lake. The rising water level forced water from the Collins River, above the dam, and through caves that emerged on a rock face of the Caney Fork River, below the dam. Since then, water has coursed through the caves. In some places, the falls are narrow drops with just a little mist. But others look like white-water springs that burst forth from the mountainside. The granddaddy of all the falls makes a 300-foot-wide, 80-foot-long drop over a

Directions

From Exit 239A, Watertown, on I-40 east of downtown Nashville, take US 70 34 miles to TN 56 south in Smithville. Turn right on TN 56 south and follow it 9 miles to TN 287. Turn left on TN 287 north, follow it 10.1 miles, then turn left into the park. The park office will be on your right after you enter the park. Continue forward 0.9 miles past the park office, and reach the Badger Flats Picnic Area on your right. The Eagle Trail starts up the hill near the picnic-area restrooms.

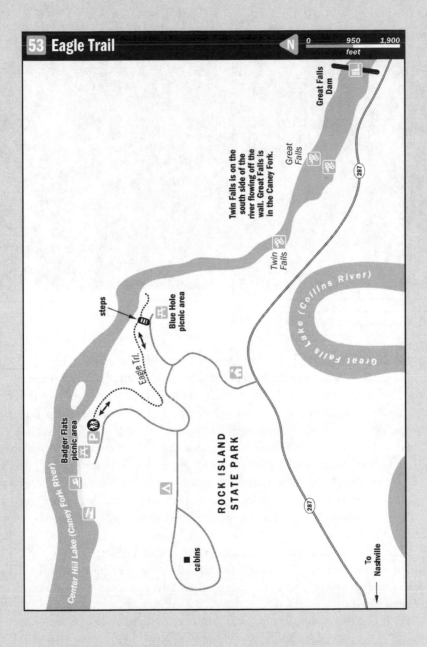

53 Eagle Trail

N

0   950   1,900
feet

Great Falls Dam

Great Falls

Twin Falls is on the south side of the river flowing off the wall. Great Falls is in the Caney Fork.

Twin Falls

287

Great Falls Lake (Collins River)

steps

Blue Hole picnic area

Eagle Trl.

Badger Flats picnic area

P

Center Hill Lake (Caney Fork River)

ROCK ISLAND STATE PARK

cabins

287

To Nashville

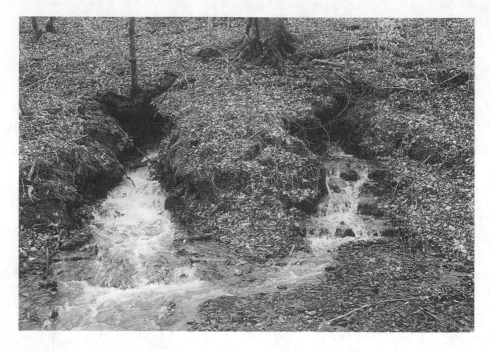

Trailside spring with a strong flow

rock bluff into the Caney Fork. This drop is known as Twin Falls. Great Falls, the lake's namesake, is actually a different cascade within the park boundaries. The Eagle Trail takes hikers by some of these unique falls. However, some gorge-scrambling at the far end of the trail is necessary to reach Twin Falls. But don't hurry because the path has a few highlights along the way.

Start the trail at the Badger Flats Picnic Area. A sign indicates that it was built under the guidance of a Boy Scout earning his Eagle Scout ranking. Pass the picnic-area restrooms and immediately enter a singletrack path. The Caney Fork River, just freed from the Great Falls Dam upstream, flows clear green against a backdrop of tan and weathered riverside bluffs. Overhead, hardwoods such as beech and hickory are sprinkled with some hemlock trees, less common in these parts. Look to your left for the last picnic table at Badger Flats. Then scramble off the path to your left and check out the first falls. Two cave openings spew water, which merges into one short stream and then falls from the riverside bluff into the Caney Fork.

Ferns dot the ground beneath the forest as the trail twists among trees near the bluff's edge; an island splits the Caney Fork River below. Past the island, the Eagle Trail turns away from the river and climbs sharply as it works around a steep and narrow feeder-stream valley. Wooden footsteps aid the climb. You will hear the sound of falling water emitting from the small valley, but it is not coming from the intermittent creek at its bottom, not in this strange place. Let your ears lead you to a small bluff in the valley, where water is emerging through caves from Great Falls Lake, which is higher in elevation than the water-emergence location.

Keep circling around the steep cove to cross the intermittent streambed on a footbridge with handrails. Come to a roadbed roughly paralleling the river to reach Blue Hole Picnic Area. Another trail leads left from the picnic area down steps of wood, concrete, and metal into the Caney Fork gorge. Here, numerous cave holes allow water to spray, foam, and descend toward the main river in multiple mini-falls. Beyond the last steps, numerous paths wrangle among the water, rocks, and trees to reach the river below. The large, flat rocks along the Caney Fork are great for sunning, swimming, and fishing.

Adventurous hikers and rock scramblers will keep upriver a short bit toward Twin Falls. Be careful, as the rocks can be slippery. The gorge is rich not only in falling water but also with wildflowers in spring.

NEARBY/RELATED ACTIVITIES

Rock Island State Park has an excellent campground, playgrounds, and game courts in addition to a boat launch and other trails. For more information, visit **www.tnstateparks.com.**

54 HIDDEN SPRINGS TRAIL

KEY AT-A-GLANCE INFORMATION

LENGTH: 4.2 miles

CONFIGURATION: Loop

DIFFICULTY: Easy

SCENERY: Cedar forests and glades

EXPOSURE: Mostly shady

TRAFFIC: Busy on weekends, moderate otherwise

TRAIL SURFACE: Dirt, rocks

HIKING TIME: 2.2 hours

ACCESS: No fees or permits

MAPS: Cedars of Lebanon State Park and Forest Trail Map, available at visitor center

FACILITIES: Restrooms, water at visitor center, picnic area at trailhead

IN BRIEF

The Hidden Springs Trail loops through a geologically interesting landscape full of rock formations and sinks, depressions in the land's surface that range from barely imperceptible wooded dips to rock fissures deeper than they are wide. Other surface features are shady thickets of cedar trees that thrive in the thin soils and cedar glades, open meadowlike areas scattered in the forest. Overall, the hiking is easy, with little change in elevation.

DESCRIPTION

This is a good hike for those who want to learn about the relationship between the land and the plants that grow on it. Also, if you want to break into a longer hike, this is it. The terrain is nearly level, and the trail remains interesting throughout. The Hidden Springs Trail is marked with white blazes painted on trailside trees. A trail sign indicates that the path is 5 miles long, but it is only 4.2 miles in length. The path crosses numerous horse trails and some old roads, so stay with the blazes and backtrack if you're unsure.

Leave the parking area and cross Cedar Forest Road. Ahead is a trail sign. The Hidden Springs Trail forks just beyond the sign. Take the right fork, as the path is easier to follow

GPS Trailhead Coordinates

UTM Zone (WGS84) 16S

Easting   0561480

Northing   3992470

Latitude   N 36° 4' 37.7"

Longitude   W 86° 19' 2.5"

Directions ⟶

From Exit 238 on I-40 near Lebanon, head south on US 231 6 miles to the state-park entrance, on your left. Enter the state park, get a trail map at the visitor center, then continue forward 1.5 miles, turning right at a park picnic area just past the park swimming pool.

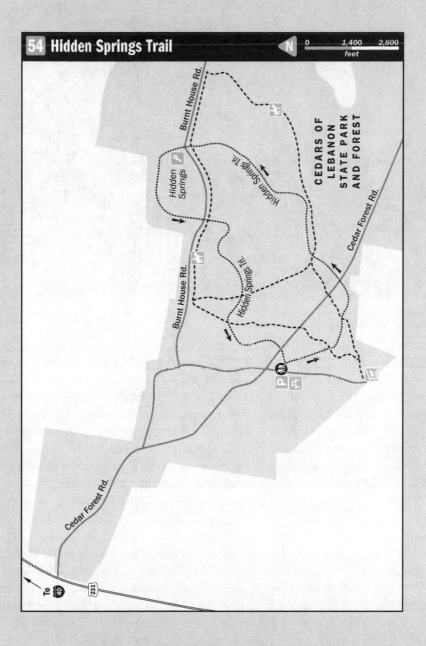

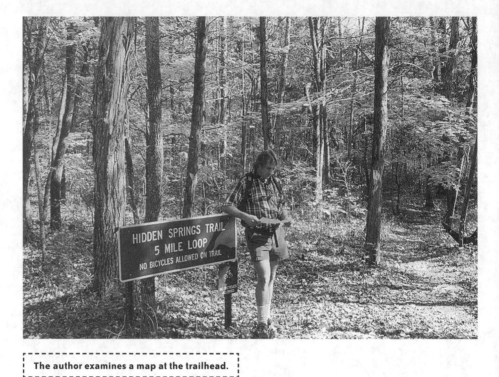

The author examines a map at the trailhead.

counterclockwise. It doesn't take long for the white-blazed path to pass by one of Middle Tennessee's signature features: a sink. These formations are caused by water erosion through caprock beneath the soil. Underground erosion continues, forming a cavern that eventually collapses and then becomes a sink. Sometimes these sinks are wide, bowl-like depressions; at other times they are deep and narrow. The numerous sinks you will see along this trail explain why there is very little permanent above-surface water here—it all runs into these sinks and into underground streams. Spur paths lead to many of the trailside sinks.

The level trail makes for easy walking among shagbark hickory, oak, redbud, and walnut, in addition to cedar trees, which sometimes grow in nearly pure stands. The forest here is broken with meadowlike clearings known as cedar glades. These clearings are natural rock gardens, albeit mostly flat, where the limestone rocks have pushed so close to the land surface that little or no soil can accumulate to allow for plant growth. In other places, where a thin soil does accumulate over the level rock gardens, the clearings may be covered with grasses or flowers. These cedar glades are a Tennessee treasure. In fact, 19 rare and endangered species of plants grow in this state and nowhere else.

Cross the first horse trail ahead. The bridle paths, identified with orange blazes, look more worn than Hidden Springs Trail, which only allows foot traffic. In places, it looks as if stones have been laid across the foot trail. Human traffic has eroded the thin covering of soil here, exposing the limestone underbelly of the forest. And sharp eyes will notice, on the left side of the trail, an old man-made pond that now functions as a wetland. Look for grasses barely covered with water.

Cross a second horse trail, then cross Cedar Forest Road at 0.8 miles. Continue forward to cross another horse trail. Notice how cedar trees grow differently depending upon their location: those in open areas, or along the edges of glades, grow robustly green down to their bases; and those in thickets (more competition for light) have dead branches at their sides and are green only at their tops. More sinks are scattered throughout the woods.

The singletrack Hidden Springs Trail winds among thickets and glades. Old wire fences indicate that this was former pastureland—poor land composed mostly of rock and thin soil. Cross Burnt House Road at mile 2.5, then reach a major sink on your right, just past a wire fence beside the trail. Walk over to this huge sink, and you will see how limbs and brush have piled against the cave opening and the water inflow of the sink. You will also notice that the spot you are standing on is overhanging the sink.

Head up along the rocky streambed that flows into this sink, cross it, and look down into a narrow fissure that keeps this streambed dry. Cross back over the streambed and come to Hidden Springs, circled by a wooden fence. This spring is actually a dug well that accesses an underground stream, which is fed by all the sinks scattered in the woods. The relationship between these sinks and streams, both above- and belowground, is complex.

Turning away from the streambed, you'll see a rock face in the middle of the woods that looks oddly out of place anywhere but in this state park. Come near the park boundary in an area of larger hardwood trees, then turn south on an old woods road to cross Burnt Woods Road again. Step over a dry streambed on a boardwalk. Pass through a pine plantation, then enter a hodgepodge of cedar glades, organized in a fashion designed only by Mother Nature. Rise into hill country, growing up in hardwoods and broken with sinkholes aplenty. Pass two horse trails in succession, then approach the Limestone Sinks Trail. A couple of side trails lead right, connecting to the Limestone Sinks Trail. Stay with the white blazes. Cross paved Cedar Forest Road, then reach the end of the Hidden Springs loop.

NEARBY/RELATED ACTIVITIES

Cedars of Lebanon State Park and Forest is a great Nashville getaway. It offers a good campground, picnic areas, picnic shelters, a lodge, and cabins. For more information, visit **www.tnstateparks.com**.

55 JOHN C. CLAYBORN MILLENNIUM TRAIL

KEY AT-A-GLANCE INFORMATION

LENGTH: 7.9 miles

CONFIGURATION: Double balloon

DIFFICULTY: Difficult

SCENERY: Lakeside forests

EXPOSURE: Mostly shady

TRAFFIC: Moderate

TRAIL SURFACE: Dirt, rocks

HIKING TIME: 4 hours

ACCESS: No fees or permits required

MAPS: Available at visitor center

FACILITIES: Restrooms, water at visitor center; picnic areas at state park

IN BRIEF

This is one of Middle Tennessee's newer trails. Laid out by the Tennessee Trails Association, it offers a rugged, challenging hike on land managed by Tennessee State Parks and the Army Corps of Engineers. Set on the peninsula of Center Hill Lake, the Millennium Trail traverses formerly settled land, rocky ridges, lakeside bluffs, and lush wooded hollows.

DESCRIPTION

This is a challenging hike, no doubt about it. When the Tennessee Trails Association laid out this path, they wanted to take hikers to all of the highlights found on this hilly shoreline of Center Hill Lake. They met their goal. But to visit all these points and stay on public land, the Millennium Trail had to make some serious twists and turns and ups and downs. It's worth every step, though. Be well rested and adventurous in spirit when tackling this trail, and then you will have a good time.

This trail is known as a double balloon, which means it takes off, makes a loop, then heads on to make a second loop. Therefore, hikers can shorten their trek, walking only the first loop if they are short on time or energy, and still enjoy this path.

The Millennium Trail leaves the park

GPS Trailhead Coordinates

UTM Zone (WGS84) 16S

Easting 0606050

Northing 3993070

Latitude N 36° 4' 42.1"

Longitude W 85° 49' 20.3"

Directions ⟶

From Exit 268 on I-40 east of downtown Nashville, take TN 96 south 3.7 miles to the park entrance. Keep forward, stopping at the park visitor center for a map. Continue for 1 mile and reach the John C. Clayborn Millennium Trail on the left.

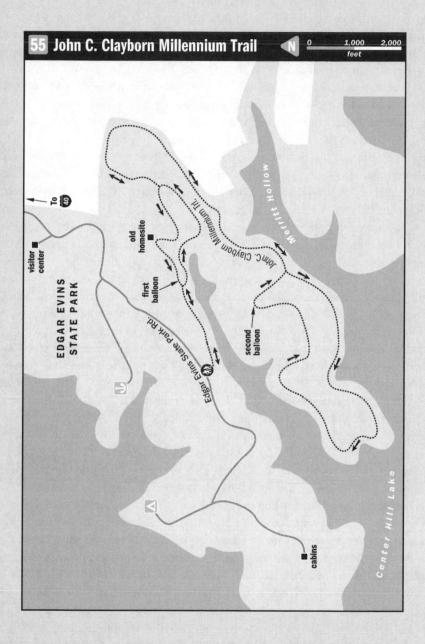

55 John C. Clayborn Millennium Trail

N

0   1,000   2,000
feet

To 40

EDGAR EVINS STATE PARK

visitor center

old homesite

first balloon

Edgar Evins State Park Rd.

John C. Clayborn Millennium Trl

Merritt Hollow

second balloon

cabins

Center Hill Lake

road and nears the shoreline before coming to the first loop, which passes by old stone walls and a homesite. The bulk of the Millennium Trail heads out for a large peninsula jutting into Center Hill Lake. The topography is rugged out here, as the path heads up a narrow hollow and gains a ridgeline by a steep but short climb. It then rides the ridge before forming the second loop, where you can gain lake views from steep bluffs.

Start the white-blazed Millennium Trail by leaving the park road and heading down an old, gated woods road into a cedar copse alongside Center Hill Lake. The embayment to your right is ever narrowing as you come alongside a stone wall. Pass through the wall at 0.4 miles, reach a trail junction, and turn right. This is the beginning of the first loop. Cross a couple of intermittent streambeds and head up a wooded hollow to reach a small flat and a second trail junction. Piled rocks indicate this little area was once tilled. The trail to your left is your return route; stay right.

Head up the hollow, which is dominated by straight-trunked tulip trees. Where the hollow dead-ends, the Millennium Trail ascends ultra-steeply to the ridgeline overlooking the hollow. Veer right and stay along the perimeter of Army Corps of Engineers land. The trail as a whole traverses both state-park and Corps property, and oaks dominate the rocky ridgeline. Reach a high knob on the ridge at mile 1.7 and gain obscured lake views through the trees. An Army Corps of Engineers survey marker is planted into the ground here. Pass a seemingly out-of-place stone wall while descending from the knob into a cedar thicket. Shortly, you'll reach a gap where a small hand-dug pond lies next to a huge oak tree with widespread branches.

The Millennium Trail descends to pick up an old woods road, then climbs to reach a gap and the start of the second loop, at mile 2.4. Stay left here and begin paralleling the shoreline on a hillside of cedar and oak, shortly stepping over a crumbling stone wall. The main body of the lake lies off to your left. Circle around a small embayment, then climb to a backbone bluffline where you can peer out on the extent of Center Hill Lake between green cedar trees.

Descend along the bluffline to reach a cliff dropping into the lake. Here, the Millennium Trail begins to curve back around the peninsula, and informal paths spur down to rocks at the water's edge. Cruise through thick woods, begin turning away from the water, and ascend the main ridgeline of the peninsula. Mostly angle up the ridgeline, until the final phase, which heads directly uphill to a gap in the ridge at mile 4.4. Once at the gap, turn left and climb on the nose of the ridge, passing another seemingly out-of-place stone wall. Meander atop the ridgeline for a half mile, then drop again to complete this far loop at mile 5.

Return to the old roadbed and backtrack 1.7 miles to reach a familiar junction in the flat with piled rocks at mile 6.7. Turn right onto untrodden trail, and trace an old farm road to shortly reach a homesite. Look for a rocked-in spring, a crumbled limestone block chimney, and foundations of an outbuilding atop the two-tiered flat. This site is a definite testimony to what was hardscrabble livin'.

Ascend from the flat, and work toward a rock pile that was undoubtedly part of the homestead just passed. Descend along a woods road to reach another trail junction at mile 7.5. Once again reach familiar terrain and backtrack the final 0.4 miles to complete the Millennium Trail.

NEARBY/RELATED ACTIVITIES

Edgar Evins State Park is a good getaway for metro Nashville. It offers camping and cabins, hiking trails, and a marina. You can choose your level of comfort or challenge here. Also nearby are outfitters that rent canoes for floating the Caney Fork River below nearby Center Hill Dam. For more information, visit **www .tnstateparks.com.**

56 JONES MILL TRAIL

KEY AT-A-GLANCE INFORMATION

LENGTH: 3.6 miles

CONFIGURATION: Figure eight double loop

DIFFICULTY: Moderate

SCENERY: Cedar glades, lake, cedar forest

EXPOSURE: Mostly shady

TRAFFIC: Heavy with bikes on weekends

TRAIL SURFACE: Dirt, roots, rocks, leaves

HIKING TIME: 2 hours

ACCESS: No fees or permits

MAPS: Available at www.tennessee .gov/environment/parks/ LongHunter

FACILITIES: None

IN BRIEF

This newer but already very popular trail in the Bryant Grove area of Long Hunter State Park was designed by mountain bikers. It travels through open cedar glades, gravel glades, and cedar forests along the shores of Percy Priest Lake. Avoid it on weekend afternoons.

DESCRIPTION

After leaving the large parking area, you'll immediately come to the first loop of the hike. Stay left here on a singletrack path, traveling the typical cedar glade woodland that comprises much of Long Hunter State Park. However, worldwide, the cedar glade is a rare environment, and we as Tennesseans should appreciate every square foot of it. The woodland floor and trail bed are quite stony, but the hickories, cedars, and oaks manage to find their place, as do boxwood bushes and moss in ultra-shady spots deep in cedar thickets.

The path runs along a hillside roughly parallel with the lakeshore below. Make a pair of switchbacks starting at 0.3 miles, then resume a northeasterly course amid trees stunted by thin, poor soil and excessive rock. Drift through open glades. At an intersection at 0.7 miles, a shortcut leads right, but the main trail continues forward in an open glade.

GPS Trailhead Coordinates

UTM Zone (WGS 84) 16S

Easting   0544133

Northing   3992131

Latitude   N 36° 4' 28.37"

Longitude   W 86° 30' 35.43"

Directions ——————→

From Exit 226 on I-40 east of downtown Nashville, take South Mount Juliet Road south 4.3 miles. Stay left at the split with Hobson Pike, traveling 1.1 miles farther to hit a T intersection and Couchville Pike. Turn left at the T onto Couchville Pike and follow it 2 miles to Barnett Road. Turn right on Barnett Road and travel 0.4 miles. Turn left into the trailhead parking.

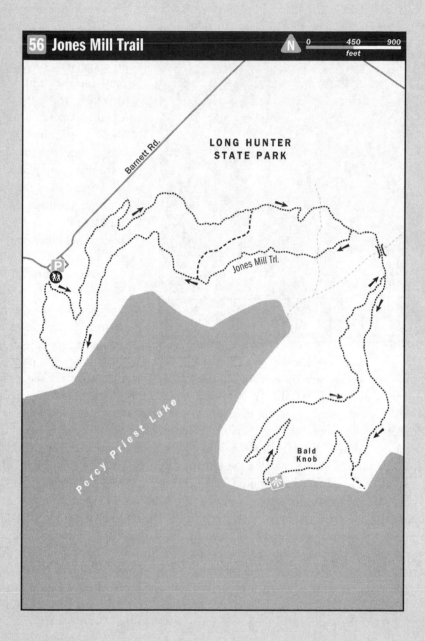

56 Jones Mill Trail

N   0   450   900
         feet

Barnett Rd.

LONG HUNTER
STATE PARK

Jones Mill Trl.

Percy Priest Lake

Bald
Knob

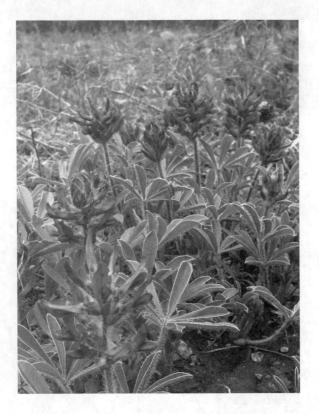

> Trailside glades fill with wild-
> flowers in spring and fall.

Note the old fence line. Woods and glades are interspersed. Be sure to stay on the trail when traveling through these open glades. Despite their appearance, they are a fragile ecosystem harboring rare plants.

Step over a wet-weather drainage at 0.8 miles. At 0.9 miles, you'll reach the other end of the first loop. That will be your return route. Keep forward toward Bald Knob to cut through a stone fence and span a drainage via a bridge. Reach the second loop at 1.1 miles—continue straight toward Bald Knob. At 1.3 miles, you may see a junction in the future, as Jones Mill Trail is being extended. Begin curving toward Percy Priest Lake in a mixed cedar forest with a grassy understory. At 1.5 miles, a faint path leads to the shore, while the main trail curves away from the lake and climbs near the crest of Bald Knob. At 1.6 miles, you'll come alongside a steeply sloped hill and shortly reach a cleared vista of the Hurricane Creek arm of Percy Priest Lake.

Switchback off the knob, still on a singletrack path, and pass through a glade at 2.2 miles and open stone slabs. Complete the Bald Knob loop at 2.5 miles, then backtrack to the trailhead loop, reaching it at 2.7 miles. Veer left into cedars and cover new terrain as you head back toward the parking area, bisecting another stone fence to pass the shortcut's south end at 2.9 miles. Wildflowers are thick here; you'll see shooting stars, phlox, and larkspur, among others. You'll pass near the water at 3.4 miles. At low water, you can access a gravel beach down here by simply aiming for the lake. The maintained trail abruptly turns away and heads toward the trailhead, which you reach at 3.6 miles.

NEARBY/RELATED ACTIVITIES

Long Hunter State Park has a lake, a fishing pier, and rents canoes and small johnboats. No gas motors are allowed, which makes for a peaceful experience. For more information, visit **www.tennessee.gov/environment/parks/LongHunter**.

OLD HICKORY TRAIL 57

IN BRIEF

This easy walk, suitable for young children, uses a combination of three mini-loops to explore the woods near Old Hickory Lake Dam. The loops traverse pine woods and go over boardwalks, culminating in a trip to a pond with a viewing platform.

DESCRIPTION

This trail is actually part of the Nashville Greenway system, though only a portion of the path is paved. The U.S. Army Corps of Engineers built it in the mid-1970s. The mounds you see in the area are part of the dredging material left from the erection of nearby Old Hickory Dam, which was finished in 1954. The forest has reclaimed the area, with the help of some loblolly pines planted in the 1960s.

Loblolly pines are not native to Middle Tennessee (they grow in a belt from east Texas to Florida and north to eastern Virginia) and are among the fastest-growing Southern pines. The pine's rapid growth makes it popular for planting and cultivation for pulpwood and lumber. Even by pine standards, the loblolly has especially fragrant needles.

 KEY AT-A-GLANCE INFORMATION

LENGTH: 1.5 miles
CONFIGURATION: 3 loops
DIFFICULTY: Easy
SCENERY: Pine and hardwood forest, willow swamp, pond
EXPOSURE: Nearly all shady
TRAFFIC: Some
TRAIL SURFACE: Asphalt, pine needles, boardwalks
HIKING TIME: 1 hour
ACCESS: No fees or permits
MAPS: Available by calling (615) 822-4846
FACILITIES: Restrooms at nearby swim beach

Directions

From Exit 92 on I-65 north of downtown Nashville, take TN 45 east 4 miles to Robinson Road, which is just after the bridge crossing the Cumberland River. Turn left on Ridgeway Road and follow it 0.5 miles to Swinging Bridge Road. Turn left on Swinging Bridge Road and follow it 1.2 miles to Cinder Road. Turn right on Cinder Road and follow it 0.8 miles to reach Old Hickory Lake. Turn left at the sign for the Old Hickory Trail, which will be on your left at 0.4 miles.

GPS Trailhead Coordinates

UTM Zone (WGS84) 16S
Easting   0530780
Northing 4016520
Latitude N 36° 17' 42.5"
Longitude W 86° 39' 24.8"

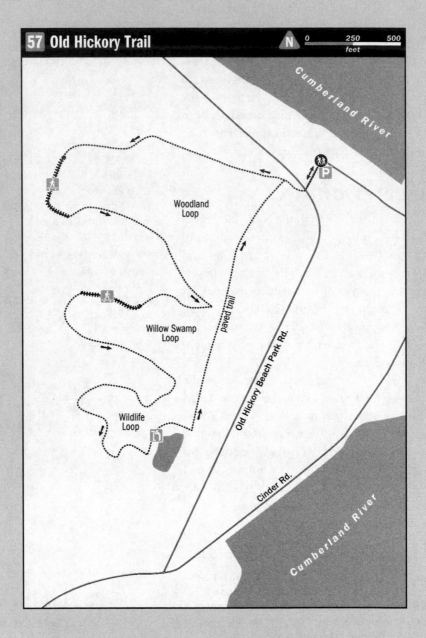

57 Old Hickory Trail

N

0   250   500
feet

Cumberland River

Woodland
Loop

paved Trail

Willow Swamp
Loop

Old Hickory Beach Park Rd.

Wildlife
Loop

Cinder Rd.

Cumberland River

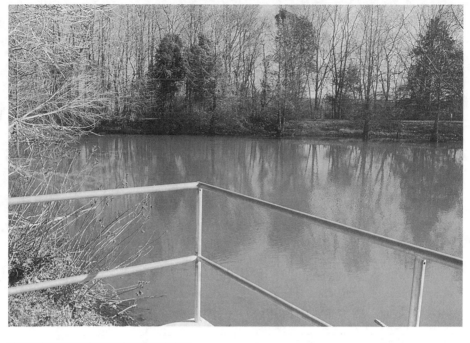

All-access pond on Old Hickory Trail

The manner in which nature repairs itself is called plant succession. For example, an area is cleared and then covered with fill. Later, plants that thrive in the sun, like blackberries, begin to grow. These species provide shade for young plants and trees that can't tolerate open sun. These trees then grow and ultimately return the forest to its former state.

Leave the parking area and soon enter the Woodland Loop. Circle through the tall loblolly pines, passing beneath a power line. A viewing blind has been built to your left. Quietly head over to the fence and peer through the boards, where a deer or squirrel may be stirring. Reach a long boardwalk that winds over a wetland. To protect them from drainage and development, wetlands have come under increasing protection over the years. Instead of viewing wetlands as useless bogs, we have come to understand them as natural filters for water as it seeps into the earth. Wetlands also foster wildlife and are a haven for insects, especially mosquitoes.

Leave the Woodland Loop at 0.4 miles, near the main paved path. Return to the woods, now on the Willow Swamp Loop. Soon reach another boardwalk. Willow trees thrive where drainage is poor, claiming their special niche in the web of life. Sycamore trees also grow along the wetter margins. In summer, the swamp emits the pungent odor of decay.

Return to the paved part of the trail, but soon turn away on the Wildlife Loop. This trail curves beneath the tall pines—notice the blackened trunks of trees here. Low-level, low-intensity forest fires often sweep through pine woods. To thrive and ultimately survive, a pine forest needs periodic fire. Some species of pine, like Florida's sand pine, need fire to open their cones.

Soon you'll emerge at a pond, where a little viewing platform allows you to peer into the water. Life at the pond varies season to season. During winter, a time of hibernation, frogs and turtles lie buried in the soil beneath the pond, and toads, snakes, and salamanders will be under old stumps and logs. Spring, though, is much more alive. Birds are singing. Ducks may be swimming. Turtles are out, enjoying the sun atop old logs. In summer, the pond may be abuzz with dragonflies chasing mosquitoes. If you come here in the evening, crickets by the thousands will be humming in harmony, and lightning bugs will be flickering off and on. Fall is when the pond will be at its lowest. Decaying leaves will be floating on the surface, later to enhance the nutrients of the pond. And marsh plants around the pond move in as the water shallows.

Follow the paved path from the viewing platform to the main paved trail. If you go to the right, the trail soon dead-ends, but you can circle the pond on an informal path. To the left, the paved trail leads through the woods past more wetlands. Enjoy this last relaxing stroll before reaching the trailhead.

NEARBY/RELATED ACTIVITIES

Old Hickory Beach is open in the warm season, is a year-round boat launch, and has picnic areas and a playground. You pass them on the way in. For more information, call (615) 822-4846.

PEELER PARK GREENWAY 58

IN BRIEF

This is a newer greenway at one of Nashville's newer parks. The asphalt path travels through a natural area of fields and woods along the Cumberland River. Toward the end, the hike makes a loop as it circles around a stream and then crosses a wetland on a boardwalk, all within the confines of lesser-visited Peeler Park.

DESCRIPTION

This hike, located near Madison, is more proof that the city of Nashville is once again turning to the Cumberland River, the reason for its location in the first place. Peeler Park is set on the inside of Neely's Bend at the end of a dead-end road. The city of Nashville first acquired the property way back in 1963, from a farmer by the name of E.N. Peeler. The city held onto the land and subsequently bought the adjacent property of Sun Valley Swim Club in 1969. For years the land was leased out as a farm. More than a generation passed before the city began to develop the park and open it for use. The resultant greenway is gaining in popularity, but the majority of users come from nearby Madison. I suggest a spring or fall afternoon to explore this little treasure that features not only the river but also a wetland

KEY AT-A-GLANCE INFORMATION

LENGTH: 2.8 miles
CONFIGURATION: Balloon
DIFFICULTY: Easy
SCENERY: Fields and woods, wetland, Cumberland River
EXPOSURE: Mostly sunny
TRAFFIC: Moderate
TRAIL SURFACE: Asphalt
HIKING TIME: 1.5 hours
ACCESS: No fees or permits
MAPS: www.nashville.gov/greenways
FACILITIES: None

Directions ————————➤

From Exit 14A (Gallatin/Madison/US 31E) on Briley Parkway on the north side of Nashville, take US 31E north to Neely's Bend Road. Turn right on Neely's Bend Road and follow it 6 miles. Turn left into Peeler Park and dead-end at the trailhead and a boat ramp on the Cumberland River.

GPS Trailhead Coordinates

UTM Zone (WGS84) 16S
Easting   0530542
Northing   4005623
Latitude   N 36° 11' 41.6"
Longitude   W 86° 39' 37.0"

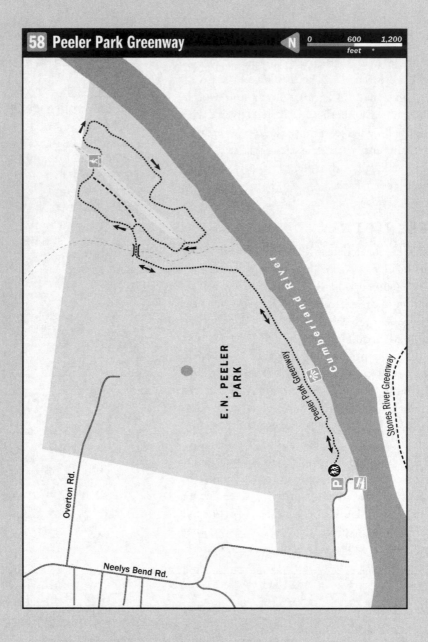

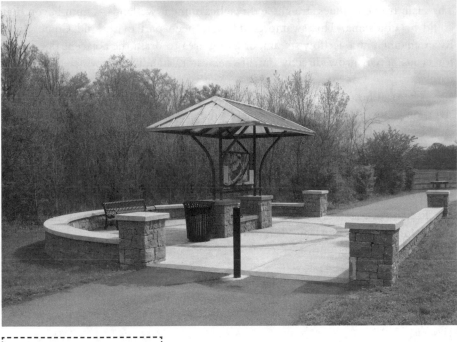

This is one elaborate trailhead.

that resembles the Deep South more than Middle Tennessee. Note: A separate set of trails is open to equestrians, but hikers and cyclists are expressly prohibited from using the bridle paths, so don't tempt fate—stick with the greenway.

Trail-users are greeted with a first-rate trailhead, complete with a shaded gazebo, metal benches, and a color map of Peeler Park. Join the asphalt track as it heads upstream on the northwest bank of the Cumberland River. A line of thick trees, cane, and brush divide you from the water about 40 feet below. To your left, a slender field runs parallel with the path. The mowed trails here are for horses, and equestrians have a separate trailhead.

Contemplation benches are scattered along the path. Travel under an open sky, walking the nexus between field and forest. Occasional spur paths lead to clearings overlooking the Cumberland. After a quarter mile, you'll reach a park-built path leading to the river. Stones River Greenway runs on the other side of the Cumberland. Peeler Park Greenway turns away from the river at 0.6 miles, now drifting into woodland bordering a tributary. The feeder stream cuts a deep ravine at this point. At 0.8 miles, the trail bridges the creek you've been paralleling, and the ravine is no longer. Shortly you'll reach the loop portion of your hike in an open area. Head left to enter canopied woods. The path is forced back toward the river as it nears the edge of the 273-acre park. At a trail junction at 1.1 miles, the wetland boardwalk is just ahead. Peeler Park Greenway was opened before the boardwalk was built, so the trail leading right was built to form a loop.

The main trail continues straight and reaches a linear wetland—a mini-bayou that could be Louisiana. This swamp could have been part of the old Cumberland River channel, an overflow stream, or a dug area to drain the adjacent floodplain for crops. Trees grow directly out of the water, standing on widely buttressed trunks.

The trail becomes paved again beyond the boardwalk. Turn back along the river, only to cross the wetland a second time in much less dramatic fashion via a culvert at 1.7 miles. Complete the loop portion of the hike at 1.9 miles and begin backtracking to reach the trailhead at 2.7 miles.

NEARBY/RELATED ACTIVITIES

Use Peeler Park as a takeout for a fantastic urban paddle trip down the Stones River from Percy Priest Dam. It is 7 miles of coldwater floating past big bluffs in a surprisingly relaxed setting.

VESTA GLADE TRAIL 59

IN BRIEF

Vesta Cedar Glade is one of Tennessee's newest additions to its state-natural-area holdings. Located on the southern edge of Cedars of Lebanon State Forest in Wilson County, this little-visited area deserves more attention. It harbors parts of the globally rare cedar glades and offers wildflowers throughout the warm season, including the federally endangered Tennessee coneflower.

DESCRIPTION

For residents of Middle Tennessee, especially southeast of Nashville, cedar glades may seem a dime a dozen. In fact, the nearest town to Vesta Glade is called Gladeville. However, when you view cedar glades and barrens from a global perspective, these plant communities are extremely rare and occur nowhere else on the planet. Even on this preserve, parts of them are fenced off from the public to limit access and protect the resource. As greater Nashville grows, these glades become developed. So, it is important that areas such as Vesta Cedar Glade be added to the Tennessee State Natural Areas program. It is also important that we visit such places, not only to personally appreciate them but also to let those

KEY AT-A-GLANCE INFORMATION

LENGTH: 1.8 miles
CONFIGURATION: Loop
DIFFICULTY: Easy
SCENERY: Cedar forests, open glades, hardwood forests
EXPOSURE: Mostly sunny
TRAFFIC: Very light
TRAIL SURFACE: Rocks and dirt
HIKING TIME: 1 hour
ACCESS: No fees or permits
MAPS: Available at www.state.tn.us/environment/na/natareas/vesta/vesta.pdf
FACILITIES: None
SPECIAL COMMENTS: There is a second, inner loop that can extend your hike.

Directions

From Exit 67 on TN 840 southeast of downtown Nashville, take the Couchville Pike east. At 0.5 miles, Couchville Pike meets McCreary Road. Continue forward from this intersection. Couchville Pike has now become Vesta Road. Continue forward on Vesta Road 1.3 miles, then turn left on Moccasin Road. Follow Moccasin Road 0.9 miles, and the trailhead will be on your left.

GPS Trailhead Coordinates

UTM Zone (WGS84) 16S
Easting 0554380
Northing 3992400
Latitude N 36° 4' 35.4"
Longitude W 86° 23' 43.9"

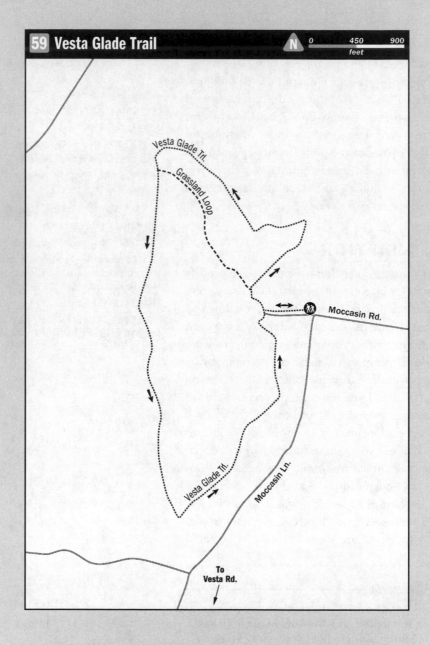

59 Vesta Glade Trail

N   0   450   900
                         feet

Vesta Glade Trl.

Grassland Loop

Moccasin Rd.

Vesta Glade Trl.

Moccasin Ln.

To
Vesta Rd.

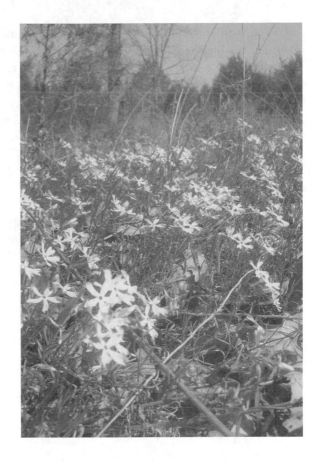

Trailside phlox brightens Vesta Glade.

who run these programs know their efforts are worthwhile.

Public access to this special area and a trail through which to walk have been a long time coming. Vesta Cedar Glade was established after the Nature Conservancy bought a 90-acre tract in 1985 and sold it to the state, which then put it under protection. Later, 60 acres of adjacent Cedars of Lebanon State Forest were added to the area because that tract also harbored rare plants, making the area a total of 150 acres.

The hiking trail through Vesta Glade passes around some boulders, heading west on an old farm road to shortly reach a junction with foot trails going in either direction. Turn right here on a narrow foot trail. The blue-blazed path winds among sinks, then opens into a glade; this is the first junction with the Grassland Loop. Stay to the right here. The fenced area you'll be bordering is the part that's off-limits to the public to protect the Tennessee coneflower. Since the state natural area's establishment, Tennessee coneflowers have been found outside the fenced area, which may seem more open than where the trail goes, because land managers are aggressively using fire and cutting invasive vegetation to improve the natural habitat for the coneflower. Other wildflowers can be seen spring, summer, and fall.

At 0.5 miles, the trail turns left and reaches a bench beneath a sizable oak by an old farm road. Continue forward here, tracing the road as it slices between a flank of cedars.

Posts with arrows help hikers keep apprised of which way to go, especially in places where vanishing-but-still-visible farm tracks crisscross the trail. This was once agricultural land, likely cattle land, and you can see fence lines and farm relics. Just ahead is the point where the inner loop, the Grassland Loop, heads through more open areas back toward the trailhead.

The path stays mostly level, but its second half becomes more canopied. Continue tracing the old roadbed until 1.3 miles. Here, the trail turns left onto a narrow track as a footpath in thick woods. Abruptly, the trail opens into a pair of gravelly glades. Watch for sinkholes bordering the trail beyond here. Just before completing the loop, pass a forgotten rock fence that likely bordered an old homesite. The settlers here probably never realized what a special place this was and that later in time the farm would be protected by the state for its outstanding features.

NEARBY/RELATED ACTIVITIES

Cedars of Lebanon State Park is north of Vesta Cedar Glade. It offers picnicking, camping, and two other hikes featured in this book—Cedar Woods Trail and Hidden Springs Trail (see pages 210 and 222).

WILDERNESS TRAIL 60

IN BRIEF

This trail, which is the most difficult trail in this entire guidebook, extends along rugged bluffs of the Cumberland River in Jackson County. The trail begins along the shoreline and climbs to the first bluff, only to descend to a steep, narrow hollow, then climb back out. This process repeats itself many times. However, your efforts are well rewarded with vistas, solitude, and a waterfall along the way.

DESCRIPTION

This trail was a real surprise. The difficulty of the trail was the big surprise, as the path literally traveled straight up and down these ravines. Its beauty was a mild surprise, with its far-reaching views from sheer bluffs cut by deep ravines cloaked in rich woods. Beauty has its price, though: technically a horse trail, the path is also traveled by hikers and only lightly traveled by both groups. The U.S. Army Corps of Engineers trail map indicates the Wilderness Trail being a loop, but nearly the entire second half of the loop is on roads. Therefore, the Wilderness Trail is best enjoyed

 KEY AT-A-GLANCE INFORMATION

LENGTH: 12 miles

CONFIGURATION: There-and-back

DIFFICULTY: Difficult

SCENERY: River bluffs, small streams, thick woods

EXPOSURE: Mostly shady

TRAFFIC: Moderate

TRAIL SURFACE: Dirt, rocks

HIKING TIME: 6 hours

ACCESS: No fees or permits

MAPS: Available at www.lrn.usace.army.mil/op/cor/rec/horseback_trails

FACILITIES: Restrooms at nearby Holleman Bend Campground

SPECIAL COMMENTS: You can make the hike 6 miles with a car shuttle on both ends.

Directions

From Exit 258 on I-40 east of downtown Nashville, take TN 53 north and stay with it a total of 17.6 miles. (At 4.2 miles, TN 53 merges with US 70N east, then diverges from US 70N after 8 more miles.) From TN 53, 17.6 miles from I-40, turn left on Holleman Bend Road and follow it 2.6 miles to a four-way stop at Ragland Lane and Forrester Hollow Lane. Turn into the campground and parking area under the big sign that says "Wilderness Trail." The Wilderness Trail leaves left from the campground to the right as you face the lake.

GPS Trailhead Coordinates

UTM Zone (WGS84) 16S

Easting 0608140

Northing 4019180

Latitude N 36° 18' 48.0"

Longitude W 85° 47' 43.9"

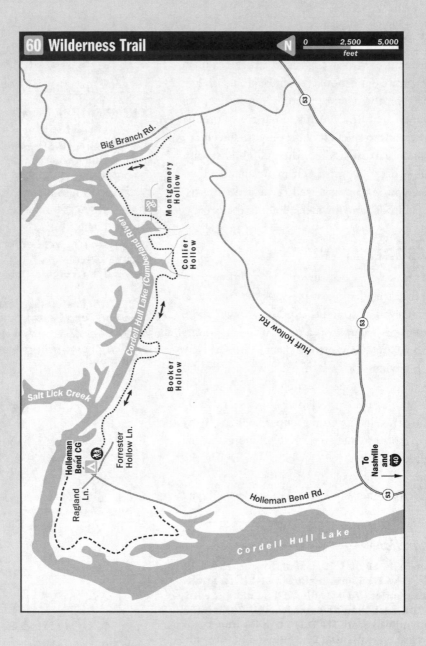

as a there-and-back hike. It is possible to put a car at the far end (directions are at the end of this narrative).

Begin the Wilderness Trail by leaving Holleman Bend Campground on the path to the right as you face the lake. This trail quickly narrows as it passes through a brushy area. Forrester Hollow Lane is to your right. At 0.1 mile, the trail turns left, passing another large trail sign and a sign warning trail travelers, "Portions of the Wilderness Trail are extremely hazardous, steep, rough, and slippery." That is all true, but careful hikers have little to fear.

Climb just a bit, then turn right on the far side of a rock wall built long before Cordell Hull Lake ever existed. The Wilderness Trail parallels the wall, then angles up to meet the crest of a river bluff at 0.7 miles. The Cumberland River, now dammed but still a ribbon of water, lies to your left. The Salt Lick Creek embayment is visible through the trees. Continue easterly along the crest of the bluff as it climbs. Watch for a side trail leading right, cutting through another rock wall to your right. This trail leads into Forrester Hollow and is part of the Wilderness Trail loop.

Mile-marker signs of various ages and types are nailed into trees alongside the path. Soon, you'll pass the mile 1 marker, reach a high point on the bluff, then descend to turn into an embayment at mile 1.5. Circle around the embayment to pass the stream flowing out of the hollow as it stairsteps into the lake. Pass another rock wall on the far side of the embayment. A little-used backcountry campsite lies trail-left before the path crosses a second streambed. Stay left here; a private trail leads right. Keep the shoreline to your left, and shortly pass the brick and concrete remains of an old homesite.

Look to your right. As the trail leaves the roadbed, it has been following and veers up a hickory-and-oak-clad hill. Top out on the hill. A sheer bluff falls to the water below, and another old stone fence runs away from the bluff. The descent from here is so steep you may be sliding on your backside before reaching the bottom. Climb just as steeply from the low point, topping out at mile 2.5. This next descent is more reasonable, but rocky, and leads to the two-pronged Collier Hollow embayment, the second major embayment along the trail. Again, circle around the embayment, stepping over a perennial stream. Open into a grassy clearing, then step over an often-dry streambed—the second prong of the embayment.

The Wilderness Trail curves along the lake and heads into another, smaller hollow, at mile 3.4. A sign advises equestrians to walk their horses through the sheer mini-gorge. The trail crosses the rocky streambed just above a wet-weather fall and climbs to circle back toward the main body of Cordell Hull Lake. Return to the bluffline and begin to circle into the two-pronged Montgomery Hollow embayment, crossing a clear stream at mile 4.1. Shortly, switchback out of the first hollow to reach a feeder stream forming the second prong of the embayment. Listen for the waterfall just upstream from the trail crossing. The low-flow cascade can be reached by simply walking up the creekbed.

Here, the path travels directly alongside the lake, before once again climbing by switchbacks toward a high bluffline. The trail then abandons the switchbacks and heads directly uphill. The route is constricted, being confined to Army Corps of Engineers property. Good views can be enjoyed through the trees along the climb, and Smith Bend of the Cumberland River and the surrounding countryside can be seen. Top out in a grassy area at mile 4.9. The drop-off here is sharp, steep, and hundreds of feet in length.

Pass a sign advising equestrians to walk their horses before making a challenging descent, then ascend through a wooded ravine. Approach a barn on private property, before dropping down a rocky bluff with mossy rocks and gnarled cedars. More views can be had while descending into the Big Branch embayment. The trail turns up the narrowing embayment in young woods before crossing Big Branch, which may be dry. Pass beneath a large sign indicating the Wilderness Trail at mile 6. At an intersection with Big Branch Road, a house is directly in front of you. To your left, downstream just a bit, is a spring and Army Corps property often used for camping. At this point, a car shuttle would be nice. Otherwise, you must backtrack.

If you choose to set up a car shuttle, back out of Holleman Bend Campground, the main trailhead, and return to TN 53. Turn left, north, on TN 53 and follow it to Big Branch Road. Turn left on Big Branch Road to reach the upper end of the embayment of Big Branch, where a large sign on the left, across from the aforementioned house, indicates the Wilderness Trail. If you have trouble finding this trailhead, just ask one of the friendly local residents, who will gladly point out the trail's end.

NEARBY/RELATED ACTIVITIES

Holleman Bend Campground is at the trailhead. It offers primitive camping, with restrooms only.

APPENDIXES
AND INDEX

APPENDIX A: OUTDOOR SHOPS

Cumberland Transit
2807 West End Avenue
Nashville, TN 37203
(615) 321-4069
www.cumberlandtransit.com

REI
261 Franklin Road
Brentwood, TN 37027
(615) 376-4248
www.rei.com

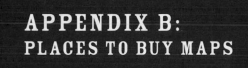

APPENDIX B:
PLACES TO BUY MAPS

Outdoor enthusiasts can find maps at the outdoor shops listed opposite; an additional resource is below.

Map Sales and Services
1100 Lebanon Road
Nashville, TN 37210
(615) 242-3388
www.mapagents.com

APPENDIX C:
HIKING CLUBS

Tennessee Trails Association
P.O. Box 41446
Nashville, TN 37204
www.tennesseetrails.org

The Tennessee Trails Association is the oldest hiking club in Middle Tennessee. The group has more going on all over the state than most hikers have time to enjoy. It is a sponsor of the Cumberland Trail and does much work in building and preserving trails and managing the wild areas of the Volunteer State.

Nashville Hiking Meetup
www.meetup.com/nashville-hiking

This Internet-based hiking group is a great place to meet fellow hikers and go hiking, among other fun activities. They hike not only greater Nashville but all of Middle Tennessee and beyond.

INDEX

A

ACCESS (hike descriptions), 3
Amulet Lake, 37
Anderson Recreation Area, 17
Anderson Road Fitness Trail, 14–17
animal and plant hazards, 8–10
Antioch Community Center, 38, 41
Artillery Monument, 192

B

Barfield Crescent Park, 162
Barfield, Frederick, 162
Barfield Wilderness Loop, 162–165
Beaman, Alvin, 100
Beaman Park, 92, 95, 100, 103
Bearwaller Gap Hiking Trail, 202–205
Bell, Montgomery, 113, 116–117
Belle Meade, 69
Bells Bend Loop, 74–77
Bells Bend Nature Center, 76–77
Betsy Ross Cabin, 45
bicyclists, best hikes for, xviii
Bledsoe Creek, 208
Bledsoe Creek State Park Loop, 206–209
Blue Hole Canoe, 38
Blue Hole Falls, 181
Blue Hole Picnic Area, 221
Bowie, Dr. Evangeline, 141, 156
Bowie Nature Park, 141, 144, 147, 156
Bowie Park Nature Center, 158
Bowie Sisters, 156
Bragg, General Braxton, 165, 188, 190
Brenthaven Bikeway Connector, 166–169
Brentwood, 166

Bryant Grove, 230
Bryant Grove Trail, 18–21
Buffalo River, 151
Buggy Hollow, 71
Burns Branch There-and-Back, 126–128
Busby Falls, 184
Busby, Thomas, 182

C

Caney Fork River, 218, 220, 229
Cedar Woods Trail, 210–213
Cedars of Lebanon State Park, 210, 225, 241, 244
Center Hill Dam, 229
Center Hill Lake, 226, 228
Cheatham Dam, 78
Cheeks Bend Bluff View Trail, 129–132
Chester Hollow, 122
children
    hikes for, xv
    hiking with, 7
city hikes, XVI
Civil War, 88–91, 165, 186–187, 190, 192
Clark, William, 148
Clarksville, 85
Clay, Henry, 196
clubs, hiking, 252
Coffee County, 182
Colbert, Chief George, 140
Collins River Nature Trail, 214–217
Concord Park, 169
Confederate Earthworks Walk, 81–84
CONFIGURATION (hike descriptions), 3
Cordell Hull Lake, 202, 204, 247

C (continued)

Couchville Lake Day Use Area, 18–21
Couchville Lake Loop, 22–25
Creech Hollow Lake, 111, 113, 114
Crockett Park, 166
Cumberland Presbyterian Church, 113
Cumberland River, 17, 37, 49, 51, 53, 55,
    237, 239, 245
Cumberland River Bicentennial Trail, 78–80
Cunningham, John, 217

D

De Montbrun, 55
Deep Well Picnic Area, 71
Defeated Creek Recreation Area, 204–205
Demonbreun Cave, 55
Devils Backbone Loop, 133–136
DIFFICULTY (hike descriptions), 3
DIRECTIONS (hike descriptions), 4
Downtown Greenway, 37
Dripping Spring Hollow, 44
Duck River, 131, 137, 174, 176–177, 181,
    199
Duck River State Natural Area Complex, 129
Dunbar Cave State Natural Area Loop,
    85–87

E

Eagle Trail, 218–221
East Fork Recreation Area, 193, 196
Edgar Evins State Park, 229
Edwin Warner Parks, 31
etiquette, trail, 10
EXPOSURE (hike descriptions), 3
Ezell Park, 41

F

FACILITIES (hike descriptions), 3
Fairview, 156
Fall Hollow Waterfall, 136
Fattybread Creek, 139
first-aid kit, 6
Fish Creek, 169
Five Mile Trail, 186–189

Flat Rock Cedar Glades and Barrens Hike,
    170–173
Forest Hills, 59
Foreword, VIII
Forrest, General Nathan Bedford, 104–105,
    123
Fort Donelson Battlefield Loop, 88–91
Fort Donelson National Battlefield, 81–84
Fort Donelson National Cemetery, 91
Fortress Rosecrans, 190, 192

G

Gallatin, 206
Ganier, Albert, 28
Ganier Ridge Loop, 26–28
Garrison Creek, 152–155
Gordon House and Ferry Site Walk,
    137–140
Gordon, John, 139, 140
Grant, General Ulysses S., 83
Great Circle Road trailhead, 37
Great Falls, 217, 220
Great Falls Cotton Mill, 217
Great Falls Dam, 214–217
Great Falls Lake, 216, 218, 221
Grinders Stand, 148

H

Hairpin Curve, 71
Hall Spring, 111
Hamilton Creek Park, 34, 48
Harpeth Hills, 29, 42, 71
Harpeth River, 116
Harpeth River State Park, 96
Harpeth Woods Trail, 29–31
Heartland Park, 64
Henry Hollow Loop, 92–95
Henry Horton State Park, 174, 177, 197,
    199
Hidden Lake Double Loop, 96–99
Hidden Springs Trail, 222–225
Highland Trail at Beaman Park, 100–103
hikes
    descriptions generally, 2–4
    east of Nashville, 200–248

southeast of Nashville, 160–199
southwest of Nashville, 124–159
west of Nashville, 72–123
hiking
    with children, 7
    clubs, 252
    recommendations (by category), xiv–xviii
    ten essentials for, 5
HIKING TIME (hike descriptions), 3
historic hikes, xviii
Hole-in-the-Wall Island, 68
Holleman Bend Campground, 247, 248
Horseshoe Trail, 141–143
Horton, Henry and John, 176, 197
Hutchins, Thomas, 169

I

IN BRIEF (hike descriptions), 2

J

Jackson, Andrew, 174, 176
John C. Clayborn Millennium Trail,
    226–229
Johnsonville State Historic Area Loop,
    104–107
Jones Mill Trail, 230–232

K

Kentucky Lake, 104, 106–107, 120
KEY-AT-A-GLANCE INFORMATION
    (hike descriptions), 3

L

Lake Barkley, 88
lake hikes, XVI
Lake Van Trail, 144–146
Lake Woodhaven, 111, 115
Lakes of Bowie Loop, 144–147
Lakeside Trail, 32–34
Lea, Luke, 69
Lebanon Pike, 64
LENGTH (hike descriptions), 3
Lewis, Meriwether, 148, 150
Little Duck River, 178, 180, 181
Little Harpeth River, 166–169

Little Swan Creek, 148–151
Loblolly Loop, 146
Long Hunter State Park, 18–21, 22, 65,
    230, 232
Louisville and Nashville Railroad, 26, 59
Luke Lea Heights, 69, 71

M

Machine Falls, 184–185
maps
    See also specific hike
    overview, map key, coordinates, 1–2
    places to buy, 251
    topo, 6–7
MAPS (hike descriptions), 3
Marshall Knob Trail, 164
McAdow, Sam, 113
McAdow Spring, 113
McCrory Creek, 63
McFadden Farm, 192
Meriwether Lewis Loop, 148–151
Meriwether Lewis Monument, 148
Metro Center Levee Greenway, 35–37
Mill Creek Greenway, 38–41
Millennium Trail, 226–229
Molloy, Johnny, ix
Montgomery Bell Northeast Loop, 108–110
Montgomery Bell Southwest Loop, 111–115
mosquitoes, 9–10
Mossy Ridge Trail, 42–45
Murfreesboro, 162, 190

N

Narrows of Harpeth Hike, 116–119
Nashville
    hikes east of, 200–248
    hikes in, 13–71
    hikes southeast of, 160–199
    hikes southwest of, 124–159
    hikes west of, 72–123
    history of, x–xiii
Nashville Chattanooga Railroad, 165
Nashville Greenway, 233
Natchez Trace, 29, 31, 137, 152
Natchez Trace National Scenic Trail, 126,
    128

N (continued)

Natchez Trace Parkway and Scenic Trail, 140
Nathan Bedford Forrest, 83
Nathan Bedford Forrest Five Mile Loop,
    120–123
National Register of Historic Places, 213
Nature Conservancy, 170, 172
NEARBY ACTIVITIES (hike descriptions), 4
Newsom's Mill Tract, 99
Nice's Mill Recreation Area, 193

O

Old Beech Bridle Path, 42, 71
Old Hickory Beach, 236
Old Hickory Lake, 206, 208, 209
Old Hickory Lake Dam, 233
Old Hickory Trail, 233–236
Old Mill Trail, 174–177
Old Stone Fort Loop, 178–181
Old Stone Fort State Archaeological Park,
    181
Old Trace-Garrison Creek Loop, 152–155
outdoor shops, 250
Overton Hills, 28, 59
Overton, John, 28
Owl Hollow Park, 31

P

Paradise Ridge, 100
Peeler, E.N., 237
Peeler Park Greenway, 237–240
Percy Priest Dam, 16–17, 64, 240
Percy Priest Lake, 14, 16, 18–20, 22, 32,
    48, 65, 67, 193
Percy Warner Park, 71
Perimeter Trail, 156–159
Pinnacle Trail, 46–48
Pioneers Cemetery, 150
plant and animal hazards, 8–10
poisonous plants, 9
popular hikes, xviii
Preface, X–XIII
Priest, J. Percy, 17
Priest Lake, 48
Purcell, Bill, 74
Pyne's ground plum, 170

R

Radnor Lake, 59
Radnor Lake State Natural Area, 26–28
Radnor Lake State Park, 57
Rattlesnake Circle, 44
Rebel Hill, 165
Revolutionary War, 210
River Park, 166
River Rats, 132
Rock Island State Park, 214, 217, 218, 221
Rosecrans, General William, 186, 190
runners, best hikes for, xviii
Rutherford County, 193

S

safety, 7–8
SCENERY (hike descriptions), 3
scenic hikes, xvi
Shelby Bottoms Nature Park: East Loop,
    49–52
Shelby Bottoms Nature Park: West Loop,
    53–56
Shelby Park, 52, 56
Sherman, General, 190
shops, outdoor, 250
Short Springs State Natural Area Hike,
    182–185
sink holes, 224
Smith, General C. F., 90
snakes, 9
solitude, best hikes for, xviii
South Radnor Lake Loop, 57–60
SPECIAL COMMENTS (hike descriptions), 3
Spring Castle, 217
Spring Hollow, 136
Stone River National Cemetery, 189
Stone, Uriah, 67, 68
Stones River, 63, 64, 240
Stones River Battlefield Loop, 186–189
Stones River Greenway, 173
Stones River Greenway of Murfreesboro,
    190–192
Stones River Greenway of Nashville, 61–64
Stones River National Battlefield, 173
Stones River Valley, 67
Swan Lake, 87

T

Tater Knob Overlook, 204, 205
Tennessee Central Railroad, 78
Tennessee Ornithological Society, 26, 59
Tennessee River, 104, 120, 122, 123
Tennessee State Natural Area, 133, 135, 170
Tennessee Valley Divide, 126, 128
ticks, 8
TRAFFIC (hike descriptions), 3
TRAIL DESCRIPTION (hike descriptions), 4
trail etiquette, 10
TRAIL SURFACE (hike descriptions), 3
trails
    See also hikes
    for bicyclists, xviii
    for runners, xviii
Tullahoma, 184
Twin Falls, 217, 220, 221
Twin Forks Trail, 193–196
Twin Springs, 34

U

UTM zone numbers, 2

V

Vaughns Creek, 29–31

Vesta Cedar Glades, 241, 243, 244
Vesta Glade Trail, 241–244
Volunteer-Day Loop, 65–68

W

Warner, Edwin, 69
Warner Parks, 42
Warner Parks Nature Center, 31, 45
Warner Parks trail system, 29
Warner, Percy, 69
Warner Woods Trail, 69–71
water, 5
weather, 4
West Fork Stones River, 162
Whitman Mill, 181
Wild Turkey Trail, 197–199
Wilderness Station, 162–165
Wilderness Trail, 245–248
wildflowers, wildlife, best hikes for, xvii
Wilhoite family, 174, 176, 197
Wilhoites Mill, 174, 177, 197
Winfry Cemetery, 107
Works Progress Administration (WPA), 213

Y

Yanahli Wildlife Management Area, 129

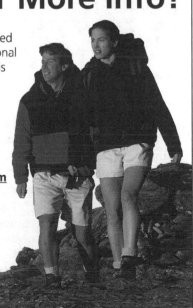
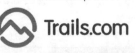

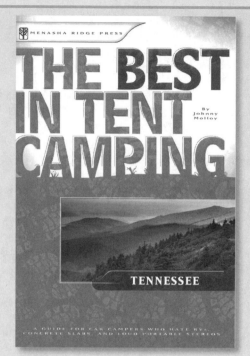

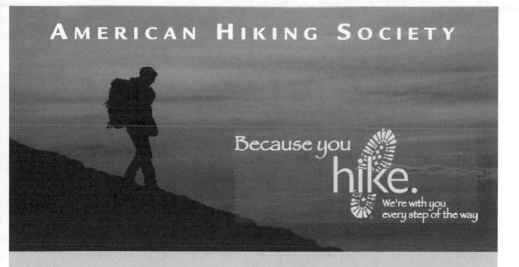
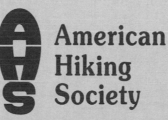

DEAR CUSTOMERS AND FRIENDS,

SUPPORTING YOUR INTEREST IN OUTDOOR ADVENTURE, travel, and an active lifestyle is central to our operations, from the authors we choose to the locations we detail to the way we design our books. Menasha Ridge Press was incorporated in 1982 by a group of veteran outdoorsmen and professional outfitters. For many years now, we've specialized in creating books that benefit the outdoors enthusiast.

Almost immediately, Menasha Ridge Press earned a reputation for revolutionizing outdoors- and travel-guidebook publishing. For such activities as canoeing, kayaking, hiking, backpacking, and mountain biking, we established new standards of quality that transformed the whole genre, resulting in outdoor-recreation guides of great sophistication and solid content. Menasha Ridge continues to be outdoor publishing's greatest innovator.

The folks at Menasha Ridge Press are as at home on a white-water river or mountain trail as they are editing a manuscript. The books we build for you are the best they can be, because we're responding to your needs. Plus, we use and depend on them ourselves.

We look forward to seeing you on the river or the trail. If you'd like to contact us directly, join in at www.trekalong.com or visit us at www.menasharidge.com. We thank you for your interest in our books and the natural world around us all.

SAFE TRAVELS,

Bob Sehlinger

BOB SEHLINGER
PUBLISHER